ILLUSTRATIONS

(between pages 38 and 39)

PELHAM

HORSEMASTER SERIES

The Horse Owner's Guide to Common Ailments

PELHAM HORSEMASTER SERIES

The Horse Owner's Guide to Common Ailments

G. W. SERTH

PELHAM BOOKS
London

First published in Great Britain by
Thomas Nelson & Sons Ltd in 1971 as part of the
Nelson Horsemaster Series

This edition published in Great Britain by
PELHAM BOOKS LTD
52 Bedford Square,
London WC1B 3EF
1977

ISBN 0 7207 1010 3

Printed in Great Britain by
Hollen Street Press Ltd at Slough, Berkshire

CONTENTS

PREFACE

This book is intended for the horse owner-groom. My object has been to describe common ailments – their nature, causes, symptoms, after-effects, treatment and (where feasible) their avoidance. Some chapters, notably that on lameness, have a preface which applies to numerous ailments in that chapter, and the reader is urged to consult this as well as the paragraphs dealing with the specific condition with which he is concerned.

My brief was to write about 'common ailments' and, with a few exceptions, those I have selected have either been seen with regularity in practice in south-east England during recent years or were shown to be common in the Survey of Equine Disease carried out by the British Equine Veterinary Association in 1962–63.

No advice urging heroic methods of treatment (such as might be useful to an owner in the outback far removed from professional help) has been given; rather have I advocated the use of tried and proven treatments with readily available medicines. As diagnosis is one of the most difficult and important aspects of veterinary medicine and surgery I urge that when simple treatments fail, professional advice be sought to confirm both the diagnosis and the treatment.

It should ever be borne in mind that the horse has a built-in repair mechanism and, in most cases, the best we can do is to help this mechanism to function. Above all do nothing to aggravate the condition. If you are not certain what to do, at least do nothing to make things worse.

When talking to Pony Club members I have told a fable about a man mending a punctured cycle tyre who suffered from a well-meaning friend. As soon as the man had applied adhesive solution to the tyre his ignorant friend washed it off with solvent; when he put on more solution his friend rendered it useless by putting on French chalk before the patch was applied. The friend knew something about tyre repairing but he did not understand it; eventually the cycle owner told his friend to go away. Moral: if you don't know what you are doing, don't interfere.

There is sometimes justification for putting sugar on wounds, but never for butter and jam. Throughout the ages ailing animals have recovered without the intervention of man – do not by ignorant interference deprive them of that chance.

Chapter 1

THE STABLE MEDICINE CHEST

Scissors	Thermometer
Forceps	Bowl
Bottle of water	Bottle of antiseptic
Cotton wool	Gamgee tissue
Gauze	Bandages
Elastic adhesive bandage	Sulphonamide powder
Acriflavine emulsion	Colic drinks
Poultices	Eye ointment
Lead lotion	Friar's Balsam

Every stable should have its medicine chest containing a few first-aid essentials. A box small enough to take to shows is an advantage. A golden rule should be that the first-aid kit should not be used for anything other than first aid: scissors which have to do double duty for first aid and mane plaiting, or bowls which are used for holding antiseptic fluid and for watering the dog are apt to be missing when urgently needed.

The equipment need not, indeed should not, be extensive. It is best to keep an adequate stock of those things regularly required and leave the more exotic items to be purchased as and when required – there is seldom an urgent call for them.

The items listed at the beginning of this chapter form the basis of a useful stable medicine chest.

SCISSORS – fairly large with blades at least 2½ in. long. If they are curved at the ends ('curved on flat') they are more convenient for removing hair around wounds. Pointed scissors are so rarely needed that it is wisest to get those with rounded blades as they are much safer when working on a restless animal. It is a good idea to attach a coloured ribbon to such items, as it makes them easier to find if dropped in straw and avoids arguments about whether or not they belong in the first-aid box.

THERMOMETER – get a clinical stub-ended thermometer, half-minute type. It is used by shaking the mercury down well below the normal temperature of the animal, lubricating the bulb (soap is excellent for this) and inserting gently for three-quarters of its length in the horse's rectum. Be sure that the instrument is in contact with the wall of the bowel and not just thrust into a ball of faeces. A horse's normal temperature is 38°C. (100–101·5°F.); it varies slightly during the 24 hours, being lowest at night and in the early morning. A rise in temperature is often the first sign of contagious disease. A common cause of very high temperature being recorded is leaving the thermometer in a hot place and forgetting to shake the mercury down before use!

DRESSING FORCEPS – a simple pair of tweezers to hold swabs of cotton wool and to remove foreign matter from wounds is a useful item. Be careful to see that they are cleaned after use and not returned to the chest with pus or other matter on them.

BOWL – plastic bowls or basins about 6 in. in diameter, such as may be obtained from any ironmonger, are suitable for holding fluid for swabbing wounds and to provide clean resting places for instruments.

WATER – a large clean bottle containing water that has been boiled is a useful item to take to gymkhanas and places where a ready supply of clean fluid may be difficult to get in an emergency. If it contains a little antiseptic it is less likely to find its way into the dog bowl or into the kettle for an emergency 'cuppa'.

ANTISEPTIC – an antiseptic is a substance which inhibits the growth of germs, it is not necessarily a disinfectant (which kills germs). Any of the proprietary brands will do, but be careful to observe the instructions regarding dilution. Antiseptics are not necessarily more effective when used in greater concentration and are much more likely to harm the tissues. Do not be misled by advertisers' claims with regard to 'healing solutions' and the like – if there is a secret to the rapid healing of wounds it lies in cleanliness and the flushing away of dirt with abundant harmless fluid at the beginning.

COTTON WOOL – buy a 1 lb. roll and when it is half used, replace it; there are plenty of other uses around the stable for the odd half pound. Cotton wool is required to carry antiseptic fluid for flushing fresh wounds and treating contaminated places. Do not be niggardly with the wool: discard it after it has been applied to a wound. Do collect your litter at shows and take it away for destruction; foxes and dogs relish tasty, used surgical swabs.

Cotton wool is also needed for applying poultices and for bandaging legs – gamgee tissue is especially useful for this.

GAUZE – if cotton wool is applied directly to a wound it is apt to stick to it and be difficult to remove later. For this reason surgical gauze should be applied in contact with wounds. It is obtainable either dry or impregnated with antiseptics or other substances. The plain variety is adequate but care should be taken to see that it is kept clean and not contaminated, and for this reason it is best to buy it in small packets. Cotton wool is usually applied on top of the gauze and the whole bandaged.

BANDAGES – half a dozen 2½ in. plain bandages are needed. They are used to hold wound dressings and poultices in place. It is not always easy to make them stay in place and a stockinette stable bandage is a useful thing to have in the first-aid chest to put on as a final covering to hold everything in position. This should be clean so as not to foul the other contents of the box or the hands of the operator, and there are obvious advantages in having it of a distinctive colour different from the others in the stable.

A roll of elastic adhesive bandage is particularly useful for holding dressings in awkward sites or when an exceptionally firm dressing is required, but if applied too tightly it may cut off the circulation and do much harm.

SULPHONAMIDE POWDER – this is one of the most commonly used dry dressings. It is dusted on to the wound after it has been cleaned, and more powder is put on a piece of gauze which is then applied to the wound, covered with a layer of cotton wool and the whole bandaged in position. Sulphonamides are obtainable on prescription from a veterinary surgeon.

ACRIFLAVINE EMULSION – can be bought without restriction and is a most effective dressing, non-stick and mild. It is applied in much the same way as sulphonamide.

COLIC DRINKS – do consult your veterinary surgeon about these. He will advise what to stock. It is important that he should know the constituents of any medicines used in first aid, as if a sick horse does not respond to emergency treatment and the veterinary surgeon has to be called in, his choice of drugs will be influenced by those already administered.

POULTICES – antiphlogistine or kaolin poultices are often needed where there is bruising, pain, or abscess formation. They can be purchased ready made. Those bought in tins should be carefully prepared according to the instructions; often they are not thoroughly heated. The tin should be opened and put in a saucepan of boiling water, as one does with a can of baked beans. Stir the contents thoroughly. It will be found that it takes a long time for the entire mass to be heated. When it is far too hot to touch, spread it in a layer about ¼ in. deep on a piece of plastic sheeting or oil-silk (the poultice has a 'drawing' effect and the purpose of the waterproof tissue is to ensure that the moisture is drawn from the flesh and not from the air). Allow this to cool until it can be borne on the back of the hand and then apply to the affected part. Cover with cotton wool in several layers to retain the heat and bandage in position. This procedure is repeated every 12 or 24 hours.

EYE OINTMENT – golden eye ointment or a sulphonamide eye ointment is the best first-aid dressing for a number of eye conditions.

LEAD LOTION – this is a useful coolant. Get a pint at a time. To use on limbs, soak a sheet of cotton wool in the lotion and bandage lightly in place. As it dries out, pour a little more lotion on the cotton wool while it is still in place on the leg.

FRIAR'S BALSAM – a few ounces of this fluid are required for steaming horses with runny noses. To steam a horse half fill a bucket with hay, pour a few teaspoonfuls of Friar's Balsam on the hay and then pour on a pint or so of boiling water. Put the bucket in a sack and use that as a nosebag to ensure that the animal inhales the steam. This is helpful to horses which have a thick nasal discharge. After five minutes add more hot water. Do not steam a horse oftener than every other day. Remember that the sack, bucket and hay are likely to be infected after use and should be dealt with accordingly.

HOOF OIL – omit this from your medicine chest. The horse's hoof is like the human fingernail and the daily soaking in oil which is the practice in some stables is as harmful to the hoofs as it would be to fingernails. Water is a normal constituent of horn and it soaks up through the horn tubules of the wall of the hoof. If these are choked with oil then the water cannot get through. In the healthy foot the only value of oil is for appearance; many horses would benefit if grooms shunned the oil bottle and spent the time saved on other grooming. That is not to say that oil is never needed, but it is the diseased hoof and not the healthy one that calls for it. On the other hand a little cod liver oil in the feed does help to promote healthy horn growth.

Chapter 2

NURSING

Proper care of an ailing horse is important in restoring it to health. Horses taken out of work should be given a light diet of hay, bran, greenstuff and the like and no corn or cubes. They should be kept warm and dry. If the coat is damp it should be dried by rubbing with hay or a rubber, and horses appear to benefit if cold ears are dried and then gently hand-rubbed from the roots towards the tips to restore the circulation.

DIET – tempt a sick horse with small amounts of appetizing food offered frequently. Clean out the manger each time before offering fresh food and ensure that nothing sour remains.

BRAN MASH – this is an excellent food for a sick horse but often it is not properly made; one must realize that a mash is, in fact, cooked. To make a bran mash put 2–3 lb. of good bran (if you can get the sort that leaves a white powder on your hand after plunging it in a sackful, count yourself very fortunate) in a clean and scalded bucket and add boiling water, stirring constantly. When the whole has been thoroughly wetted (with 2–3 pints of water) wrap up the bucket in a horse blanket or several sacks to conserve the heat and allow it to cool slowly; this takes several hours.

Bran mashes can be made more palatable by adding an ounce of salt or a few crushed oats, providing the horse is not suffering from a disease in which these must be avoided.

LINSEED MASH – this is made by adding 1 lb. of prepared linseed to a bran mash. The linseed is prepared by simmering in about four pints of water for several hours until a jelly is formed. It is important that the water should be kept almost at boiling point because linseed sometimes contains a substance (a cyanogenic glucoside) which when activated by warm water produces the highly poisonous prussic acid. However, this is destroyed when the temperature of the water is raised to boiling point for an hour or two.

WATER – horses do not enjoy warm water and even in cold weather the drinking water should only be heated to about 10°C. (50°F.).

VENTILATION – fresh air is always required and there need be no fear about allowing a horse to have plenty of it, but draughts must be avoided. If the animal is cold and shivery put on adequate clothing but avoid making the patient uncomfortable by over-clothing. A layer of straw put on the back under the rug helps to keep the heat in, as does the use of a cellular sweat sheet.

STABLE CARE – if the horse is kept in the stable for some days, care should be taken to prevent the legs from filling by applying stable bandages and hand-rubbing the limbs night and morning when the bandages are changed. This should be at least night and morning.

Do not over-fuss a sick horse: grooming may well be restricted to wiping over with a damp sponge.

In all cases, but especially where there is infectious disease, be clean. Infected dressings and discharges are best burnt.

A loose box is preferable to a stall for the sick horse, and if artificial heat, such as an infra-red lamp suspended from the ceiling, is provided so that the amount of clothing can be reduced, the animal will be more comfortable.

As certain treatments are referred to several times in later chapters, to avoid repetition a description is given of them here.

TUBBING – this is the treating of the horse's foot with hot water which usually contains a little antiseptic. The foot should first be well washed and scrubbed. It is then soaked in a bucket or bowl – plastic utensils are best as they are less apt to clatter and frighten the animal. The water should not rise above the level of the hoof and it should be hotter than one can comfortably bear on one's hand. As it cools more hot water should be added, taking care, by discarding some of the old, that the fluid does not rise above the top of the hoof. If the higher parts of the leg are being treated then the water should be cooler, as hot as one can comfortably bear oneself, and it should be splashed or sponged on to the affected part. The treatment is applied two or three times a day for 20 minutes or half an hour at a time. Tubbing is often followed by poulticing.

COLD HOSE – this is a valuable first-aid treatment in many limb injuries. Special equipment is available that can be fastened round the limb and attached to a hose. Perforations in the device allow the water to escape all round the limb. In the absence of such an apparatus home-made contrivances can be quite effective. The cooling effect depends largely upon the evaporation of the water, so a gentle stream will cool more quickly than a violent jet. If no hose is available it may be possible to rig up a large container above the horse and by means of a piece of tubing allow the water to trickle on to the leg. Failing such methods, a cloth soaked in cold water and wrapped round the limb is quite effective, especially if it is in a current of air. Again remember that it is the evaporation rather than the initial coldness of the water that produces the required effect.

Generally the best results with hose piping are obtained when the water is left running on the limb continuously, but failing this even 20 minutes or so a day will often help.

MASSAGE – very light rubbing with the fingertips has an easing effect on painful conditions. When the pain is less severe but the part is swollen the excess fluid in the area may be encouraged to disperse by firmer pressure with stroking movements towards the heart. Unless a lubricant such as soap and water or liquid paraffin is used, however, the friction may inflame the skin.

HORSE UNABLE TO RISE – a not infrequent happening is that a horse lies down in its stable and gets into such a position that it is unable to rise, as when the animal's legs are under the manger, or when a foot becomes trapped under a stall division. Such a horse is said to be 'cast'. Should this happen it is essential to take things calmly and not to excite the horse, causing it to struggle and so

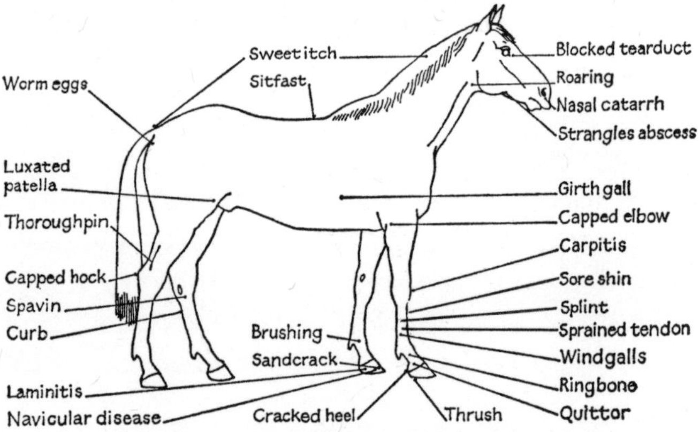

Fig. 1 Seats of Common Ailments

make things worse. Remember that the horse, although lying quietly, may suddenly plunge endangering anyone who is near. Put a head-collar on the animal and, if possible, push a sack filled with straw under its head; this acts as a pillow to prevent injury and discourages the horse from rising – as all circus trainers know. The horse's reflex mechanism causes it to try to rise when its head is pressed down but it will stop trying to get to its feet if its head is raised slightly. It may be possible to manipulate the feet free and enable the animal to rise; if this has to be done it is safer to move the legs with ropes than to stand close and move them with one's hands. At other times it is necessary to put ropes under the animal and drag it bodily away, and in some cases it may even be necessary to cut away obstructing woodwork. Get the horse into a position from which it can extend its forelegs and raise itself head end first. Then extend the limbs into the rising position. If the horse has been down for some time it may be cramped, in which case you should roll it on to its other side and massage the limbs before trying to make it get up.

Chapter 3

LAMENESS

All who study the anatomy of the horse must be impressed by the complex and effective mechanism for the avoidance of shock transmission. In the foot there is the elastic-walled hoof, the soft springy frog and the pedal bone, supported as it were in a fluid bath of blood with the lateral cartilages affording a further shock-absorbing mechanism. At the fetlock there is an angled joint which hinges when weight is put on it. Each joint in the limb has cartilage covering the ends of the bones and the whole is surrounded by lubricating fluid in the elastic bag called the joint capsule. Higher up the limb we have the permanently angled elbow and shoulder joints, while the shoulder blade itself, the topmost bone of the foreleg, has no bony connection with the trunk but is connected by muscles which take up much of the residual shock passing along the limb. The complexity of the shock-absorbing mechanism points to the importance nature places upon the absence of jar. When man comes to use the animal for riding he tends to increase the concussion and jar and to eliminate some of the natural shock absorbers. Thus he adds to the weight that has to be borne, he induces the animal to go at fast paces

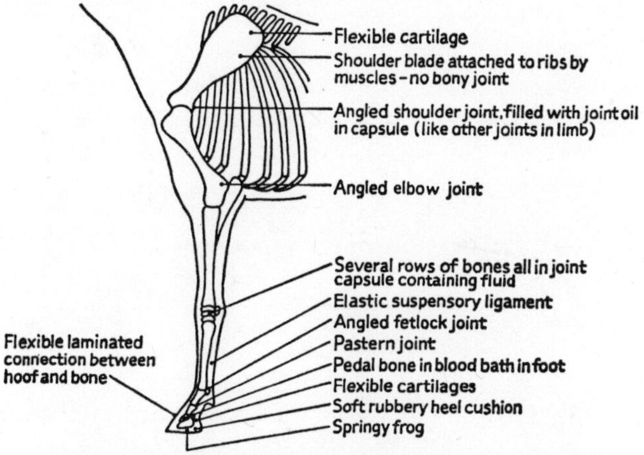

Fig. 2 The natural anticoncussion mechanism of horse's foreleg

on unnaturally hard ground, and he prevents the function of the frog and the expansion of the hoof walls by the use of iron shoes. As would be expected, those structures which nature takes such elaborate precautions to protect suffer when abused in this way, and such ailments as splints, sore shins and ringbone can be caused. These similar diseases, similarly caused, have in many cases similar treatments.

The young horse with its undeveloped limbs has only a light body to carry. The growing bones are even less capable of enduring abuse than are the limbs of an adult animal. Thus it is that these ailments most frequently affect the young horse when it is first put to work, required to carry a load, and ridden fast on hard going. It is well known that early backing of young racehorses may lead to spinal damage with fusion of the vertebrae, as well as to disease of the limbs.

The detection of lameness is not always easy. In severe cases where the animal holds up or rests the injured limb the identification of the injured member is simple, but location of the precise site and then diagnosis of the

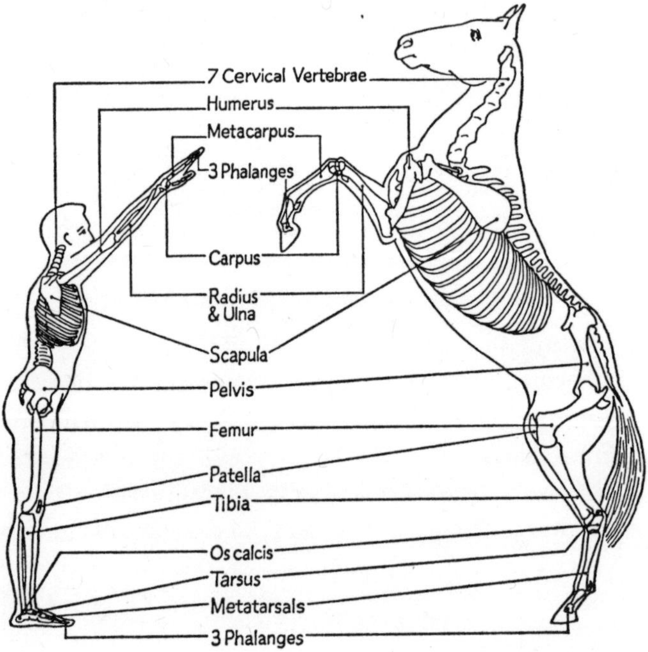

Fig. 3 Skeletons of horse and man compared

disease may present many problems. Most lameness is more pronounced at the trot than at any other pace, and the rule is that the horse raises its head when a painful fore-limb comes to the ground and drops its head as the sound foot takes the weight. If the lameness is in a hind limb then the horse tends to drop its head as the injured limb comes down as the weight is thus taken on the foreleg and the hind limb is relieved. Some lameness is more obvious when the horse is circled. If a foreleg is painful then lameness below the knee will be accentuated when that limb is on the inside of the circle, while the lameness from pain above the knee tends to be shown more when that leg is on the outside of the circle. Most lameness in the foreleg is below the fetlock, and in the hind limb the hock is the commonest site of lameness.

For more precise location of lameness veterinary surgeons employ regional anaesthesia, injecting a solution of local anaesthetic on the course of a nerve and so removing sensation from the parts supplied by it. If the horse then goes sound it indicates that it no longer feels pain and the lameness lies below the site of injection.

X-rays, too, are a valuable aid to diagnosis of lameness. However, useful though the radiograph may be, it is not, unfortunately, the answer to all our diagnostic problems, which still call for the skill of the trained hand and eye.

SHOULDER LAMENESS – This is included for the sake of completeness, but when dealing with riding horses shoulder lameness is not a common ailment. 'Sweeney', atrophy of the muscles due to paralysis of the suprascapular nerve caused by pressure from an ill-fitting collar, was fairly common among young plough horses, but otherwise lameness arising in this region is infrequent, except when due to a blow.

CAPPED ELBOW – Persistent irritation or injury to the elbow causes the condition of capped elbow, or 'shoe boil' as it is often called because of its commonest cause. This is a soft swelling over the point of the elbow, at the back of the leg about on a level with the under line of the horse's chest. The swelling fluctuates and may or may not be painful. Sometimes it causes lameness. Some horses when lying down tuck the foreleg under themselves in such a way that the heel of the shoe contacts the elbow, and it is this persistent irritation that gives rise to capped elbow.

The condition can be avoided by careful shoeing to avoid the iron projecting or by the use of a 'sausage boot', which is a thickly padded strap which one affixes to the pastern when the horse is stabled. The pad is so large that it prevents complete flexion of the joint and so keeps shoe and elbow apart. Insufficient bedding can also result in capped elbow.

The most important part of treatment is removal of the cause. Early cases will respond to cold applications. More chronic cases call for the use of a mild blister, while infected 'boils' may need treatment with antibiotics or surgical opening and drainage.

SORE KNEES – Injury to the knee by strain or blow causes inflammation which is known as carpitis. The condition is painful and the horse is markedly lame. The knee becomes swollen and the animal resents the joint being pressed or flexed. In the early stages apply loose cold water bandages, cold hose, or astringent lotions on a compress. Hot applications in the form of poultices will help once the acute inflammation has subsided. In the more serious cases it may be necessary for a veterinary surgeon to draw off the fluid and inject anti-inflammatory drugs such as corticosteroids.

SORE SHINS – This condition is most commonly seen in young racehorses starting work and is due to concussion injuring the periosteum (membrane covering the bone) on the front of the cannon bone. The affected animal is very lame and in much pain. The front of the cannons are swollen and tender to the touch. Treatment comprises rest and cold applications. Complete recovery is the rule unless heroic treatments have been rashly applied.

SPLINTS – Splints are one of the commonest ailments of the riding horse and provide another example of 'concussion' lameness. The main bone of the limb below the knee or hock is the metacarpal (metatarsal in the hind limb) or cannon bone. On each side of this is a very much smaller bone called a splinter or splint bone. These splint bones take part in the formation of the knee or hock joint at their top ends but do not extend down the limb all the way to the fetlock joint. The splint bones are bound to the cannon bone by fibrous tissue and in the young horse some movement can occur between the bones. As the horse grows older the fibrous tissue changes to a bony union and the three bones become fused into one. If, while the fibrous tissue still exists, it is strained it may tear slightly (the heads of the splint bones form the inner and outer parts of the knee joint and the hock, and anything which causes the strain to be off-centre, such as stepping on an irregular surface, deformity of a limb or a failure in co-ordination can strain the limb in this way). To repair the damage, nature causes inflammation to take place with the usual pain, swelling and heat of the affected part. The horse will become lame and the signs of inflammation can be detected on the inside or outside of the cannon bone, but more commonly on the inside because the bone formation of the knee tends to put greater weight on the inner bone. This inflammation will be followed by a hastening of the deposition of bone in the fibrous tissue and a solid union between the splint bone and the cannon bone. Usually more bone is deposited than is required and a lump known as a 'splint' is formed. If the horse is worked before the splint has been completely solidified more damage may occur and an even larger lump ensue. X-rays are of great value in determining the type of damage and therefore of treatment required. Splints may be hereditary and occur without any apparent excitatory cause.

Treatment consists of rest and the application of cold lotions to the part to ensure that the inflammation is not excessive. An old treatment was to cut a hole in a piece of sole leather, fit the lump into the hole and then bandage tightly to lessen the blood supply to the part, and sometimes a piece of lead was used in a similar manner. It is improbable that these treatments hastened return to work more than the conservative methods described. When bone has been laid down to unite the splint bone and the cannon bone, further movement is inhibited and unless such excessive strain is applied to the limb that this bony union breaks down fresh splints on the affected bone are unlikely. Consolidated splints usually cause no trouble unless these are so large, or so sited, as to impinge on and interfere with the functions of other structures. Firing and blistering are sometimes used on recalcitrant lesions. Mineral supplements to the diet may be called for. (An enlargement on the cannon bone clear of the splint bone and usually due to a blow is called a 'bump'.)

SPRAINED TENDONS – Inflammation of tendons is known as tendinitis and is most commonly due to sprain. The function of muscles is to cause joints to flex and extend. The muscles are attached to bones by fibrous tissue; when this tissue is in the form of a cord it is known as a tendon. In the horse the word 'tendon' is generally used to refer to the tendons which unite the large muscles above the knee and hock with the bones below these joints. Oddly enough, horsemen employ the term 'bone' to indicate the circumference of the cannon, a mass of tissue which includes bone, the tendons, blood vessels, nerves and connective tissue.

Tendons are strong and usually only give trouble when very excessive strain is thrown on them. This occurs when the horse makes a move of faulty co-ordination as happens when the going changes suddenly from hard to soft or vice versa, or when a great recovery effort is made, or when a tired or ill-conditioned animal suddenly exerts greater effort; this last factor is probably the most important. Muscles work in pairs, so that one opposes the other, one flexing a joint and the other straightening it. A lack of co-ordination between these pairs can result in a strain. Bad shoeing has also been implicated, and poor conformation, as well as the practice of training a horse when too young, may easily lead to tendon sprain.

Sprained tendons are very serious and no risks which might give rise to them should be taken.

Tendinitis causes pronounced lameness. The affected

parts are swollen and painful and the animal rests the limb in such a position as to relieve pull on the injured tendon.

Old sprains of the tendon may be recognized by the back line of the tendons being bowed. Such animals are said to have 'sprung' tendons.

Even the mildest cases should be regarded gravely, and it is as well to accept the fact that any case of sprained tendons is likely to put the horse out of action for the rest of the season.

Nature is apt to be over-exuberant in her repair methods for tendons, and the immediate use of cold applications from a hose, or of refrigerant lotions, is indicated. These will reduce the supply of blood to the part, lessen pain and swelling and make the formation of adhesions between the tendon and its sheath less likely. The swelling that ensues from a sprained tendon is due to fluid which accumulates in the part, and this can be kept away by the application of tight bandages over cotton wool. Care should be taken to see that the cotton wool protrudes beyond the top and bottom of the bandage. If a sheet of cotton wool or gamgee tissue is wrapped two or three times round the leg and held in place with a tight bandage another stable bandage can be placed on top of this and pulled as tight as possible without fear of damage. If the swelling in the leg is insufficient to obliterate the grooves between the tendons and the cannon bone, these grooves should be filled with cotton wool rolled into a cigar shape, so that the pressure on the tissues is equalized. It is wise to have further bandages and cotton wool ready when removing pressure bandages so that they can be replaced with the least delay and thus avoid fluid filling the tissues while the bandages are being changed. Pressure bandages should be replaced at least twice daily.

Rest is advocated until the severe symptoms have abated. The horse should, of course, be put on a light diet with no corn. Once these symptoms have subsided, usually in a day or two, massage will help to remove the fluid and prevent the formation of adhesions. A lubricant such as soap and water or liquid paraffin, or a mild embrocation such as soap liniment, should be used so that the skin is not irritated by friction. Massage is helpful in most cases, even the advanced chronic ones.

Movement is also advisable to prevent adhesions. In the early stages this can be passive, the attendant flexing the knee by raising the affected leg and then gently easing the foot towards the elbow. The horse is likely to resent this at first but with gentle manipulation will usually allow the limb to be bent more and more. As the condition eases, exercise in hand should begin, and be increased in duration each day. Finally, the horse should be turned out to grass where this is practicable. The gravity of a case of sprained tendon will depend upon the amount of damage done by tearing to the tendon and its sheath. If it is very severe there may never be recovery, even to the stage of light work.

More drastic treatment is needed in severe cases, and a modern treatment consists of severing the tendon in a longitudinal direction under local anaesthesia to induce an increased blood supply in the chronic stage of the disease. Line, point, and acid firing and blistering all have their advocates and the writer has seen good results attend the use of a special boot containing coiled springs which exert pressure on the injured parts. Tendon transplants are now used in selected cases.

WINDGALLS – Soft synovial swellings just above and behind the fetlock joint are known as windgalls. There are two types: tendinous and articular. Where the tendons pass behind the fetlock joint they are enclosed in a sheath containing lubricating fluid (synovial fluid) and strain results in the production of more fluid which causes the sheath to swell. If the strain is of the fetlock joint then the excess fluid will cause the joint capsule to bulge, forming an articular windgall. These swellings are very common, usually painless and, apart from unsightliness, of little significance except in young horses. Stimulation of the skin over the swellings by the use of rubefacients, such as liniment or mild blisters, will often cause a decrease in the size of the windgalls, as will pressure bandaging after work. Surgical aspiration of the fluid followed by the injection of substances to destroy the secreting membrane or reduce inflammation is less successful than might be hoped.

INTERFERENCE – A frequent cause of extreme lameness is the striking of one limb by another ('interference'). Most commonly this is in the fetlock region and it is then called 'brushing'. A horse going sound one moment is suddenly acutely lame and may even refuse to put the injured limb on the ground. When the interference is high, just below the knee, as happens with high-actioned horses, it is called 'speedy-cutting' and in extreme cases an animal may fall as if shot. Rest and cold-hosing are indicated.

RINGBONE – Ringbone is the term used to describe the deposition of extra bone on the first or second pastern bone, or on both. It is most common in the forelegs and is due to injury such as a blow or sprain or concussion. Veterinary surgeons distinguish between 'true' ringbone involving the joint between the two pastern bones and 'false' ringbone which is on the shaft of the bone, and they attach an even gloomier prognosis to the former than to the latter.

An affected animal is lame and the bone concerned is enlarged and the area swollen. Except in advanced cases X-ray examination may be needed to confirm the diagnosis. In the early stages reduction of the inflammation by cold applications is called for and rest for several months is imperative. If the case is discovered early, it is possible that the inflammation (which is followed by deposition of bone on the affected area) will be localized. However, if so much bone is laid down that the joint between the two pastern bones is affected, then permanent lameness is likely. Even the ground in a field during the summer may be firm enough to aggravate the condition if the horse moves quickly, and should the going get very hard then restriction of movement in a stable or yard is required. Firing is sometimes necessary.

FRACTURES – The popular belief that a broken bone always means that the horse has to be destroyed is far from the truth. When dealing with fractures in the horse many special difficulties arise that do not occur in man, including the great weight and strength of the animal which may make splinting ineffective, the problem of 'bed rest', the cost of certain techniques when compared with the value of the animal and the expense of protracted stabling for an idle animal. In addition to these problems there is the fact that, generally speaking, nothing less than complete recovery of function and usefulness can be regarded as satisfactory. A horse with a 'mechanical lameness' may still be useful at stud but potential breeding animals form only a small proportion of those at risk.

Notwithstanding the difficulties, many fractured bones can nowadays be restored to useful function. Mainly this is due to progress in 'internal fixation' – by which is meant the application of metal plates screwed directly on to the bones – and other methods of holding the fragments together, such as screws and metal pins. Of course, these techniques can only be used in veterinary hospitals and it goes without saying that professional advice should always be sought where a broken bone is feared.

A fracture should be suspected when there is angulation in a part of the limb that is normally straight, a grating sensation when the limb is moved and the broken parts rub together, pain, swelling, and an unwillingness to put the limb to the ground. What is known as a 'star' fracture sometimes occurs when a horse receives a kick from another animal. The injured bone is not broken in two but 'stars' much as a thick window does when struck by a stone. In such a case the bone is so weakened that movement may result in complete breakage.

First aid should comprise keeping the horse still until professional aid arrives. Movement, such as attempting to get the horse into a box or vehicle, may change a reparable fracture into a hopeless case. If circumstances necessitate movement of a horse with a broken leg a splint can be devised from two pillows, two broomsticks, and some stable bandages. Bend the pillows round the affected limb and fasten in place with tight stable bandages. Put a broomstick on each side of the leg and bind these to the pillows with more stable bandages.

Of course, limb bones are not the only ones liable to fracture. In many cases where other bones are broken the fractured pieces may be removed surgically and the animal suffers no loss of usefulness.

It may be some consolation to the average horse owner to know that by far the highest number of fractures occur in racehorses.

LAMINITIS – This condition, also known as fever in the feet or founder, is a frequent and often avoidable condition. It is commonest in ponies, but can occur in any type of horse. It may involve any foot or all four. There are many causes, the most frequent being over feeding, especially with protein-rich foods, as when a greedy horse gains access to the corn bin. It may also arise when a horse is idle following systemic disease, from ingestion of cold water by an overheated animal, or concussion from hard, fast road work.

The sensitive laminae in the feet which engage with the horny laminae of the hooves become inflamed and engorged with blood. The horse is in great pain and the condition might be likened to a person wearing a tightly laced boot and developing a boil on his foot, yet being unable to undo the lacings to relieve the pressure. The forefeet are most commonly affected and the patient will adopt a typical stance with the hind feet drawn up under the body and the forefeet extended forward so as to relieve them of weight. The animal is most reluctant to move forward, it may perhaps be down and refuse to rise. There is usually a high temperature.

Treatment consists of a light diet of hay and bran, a purgative such as Epsom salts in a bran mash, and cooling the feet by either standing in a stream or in wet mud, or by applying cloths soaked in cold water. Exercise will increase the drainage of blood from the feet but may cause such pain as to be inhumane; in such cases veterinary surgeons sometimes block the nerves to the feet with local anaesthetics and then exercise the horse while the feet are numb. There are several new and highly effective drugs used by the veterinary profession for laminitis.

Prompt treatment of this disease is important. If it is neglected the connection between the sensitive and insensitive laminae of the feet may be loosened and permit the pedal bone (third phalanx) to rotate and, in extreme cases, to penetrate the sole of the foot. The description given applies to 'acute' laminitis, but there is a form known as 'chronic' laminitis which may follow the acute type or come on slowly without acute symptoms being shown. In this form the wall of the hoof usually shows pronounced rings around it – where the growing horn has been pushed out by the displaced bones inside the hoof – and the animal is slightly lame.

Special shoeing may be needed in cases of laminitis.

NAVICULAR DISEASE – The description navicular disease is one of the dread lamenesses and usually affects horses of seven years of age or more that have worked on hard

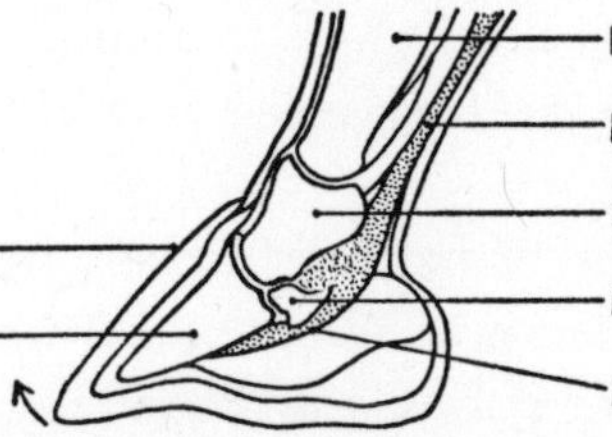

Fig. 4 When toe is long, raised in direction of arrow, extra pressure is put on the navicular bone by the deep flexor tendon at X

going. It is a name given to several types of disease which affect the navicular bone (shuttlebone) which lies between the flexor tendon and the third phalanx (pedal bone). Nearly always it is the forefeet which are affected. The lesions on the navicular bone may take the form of ulcers, bony out-growths (osteophytes), calcium deposits or change in the structure of the bone.

The actual cause is unknown but concussion and excessive strain in hunting and jumping seem to be important factors. When pressure is put on the tendon, as in landing from a jump, the navicular bone is squeezed. The longer the toe of the foot the greater the pressure. Overlong feet will cause constant pressure, as opposed to the intermittent pressure caused by the contraction of the muscle pulling on the tendon. If the horse is constantly working on hard ground such as paved roads then the damage inflicted on the navicular bone is likely to be greater than if the going is resilient as it is on grass. It is not surprising, therefore, that this condition is commonest in horses badly or infrequently shod and doing much road work. There are other factors involved in the production of this disease including heredity, feeding, and the nature of the soil on which the animal was reared, but there is no doubt that the shoeing factor is one of the most important.

The symptoms of navicular disease are insidious in onset. At first there is only a suspicion that something is wrong and on examination the animal may appear to trot sound. But sooner or later the telltale 'pointing' will begin and the horse when resting will be seen to put one foot in front of the other and rest the foot on its toe, thus relieving the pressure on the navicular bone. This pointing of the forefeet is characteristic of navicular disease but it should be remembered that it only applies to the forefeet – it is usual for a healthy horse to rest its hind legs in this manner. As the disease progresses the horse becomes pottery in its gait and tends to stumble. The feet gradually change shape and become contracted at the heels. If the horse is made to stand its foot on a plank which is then raised at the front end so as to bend the toe upwards and thus put strain on the tendon over the navicular bone it may show pain and go more lame than before.

Generally the lameness is most marked when first beginning work and then wears off, but as the disease progresses lameness becomes continuous.

Treatment of navicular disease is usually unsatisfactory. Steps should be taken to reduce concussion by the use of leather or plastic pads under the shoes, by keeping off hard going – at least at the faster paces – and, where there are osteophytes, by allowing more room in the foot by grooving the walls of the hoof and encouraging it to expand. In other cases injections to encourage adhesions to the bone are used with success. Usefulness (at any rate for a time) may sometimes be restored by the operation of unnerving (removing a section of nerve conveying sensation from the foot) – an operation that is, however, accompanied by disadvantages.

PEDAL OSTITIS – This is inflammation of the third phalanx (pedal bone) in consequence of which inflammation, bony outgrowths (osteophytes) form on the pedal bone. These press on the sensitive laminae and often cause great pain and lameness. Again, concussion is one of the main factors in the production of this disease.

Lameness tends to disappear and then recur with increasing severity and finally become permanent. Pain in an acute case can be relieved by rest and cold foot baths. Surgical shoeing may be needed.

If lameness persists after taking these measures, grooving the wall of the hoof and avoiding work causing concussion, the only alternatives left may be unnerving or slaughter on humane grounds.

BRUISED SOLE AND CORNS – Bruising of the sole is caused by stones and rough going and is commonest in horses with flat feet and thin soles. When the bruise affects the sensitive tissues at the angle of the wall and the bar of the foot it is known as a 'corn'. Corns are frequently caused by bad shoeing or leaving the shoes on too long so that they 'grow into' the feet. Shoes which are too short or fitted too close tend to cause corns. The commonest site for corns is the inner heel of a forefoot. It is for this reason that a farrier, when removing a shoe, usually puts his pincers first under the outer heel, so avoiding pressure on the 'seat of corn'.

Corns are known as 'dry' when there is not much to see but the reddish discoloration of the horn from effused blood; 'moist' when the injury has been more severe and the tissues are sodden with effusion; and 'suppurating' when there is infection. This last type of corn may, in addition, involve surrounding structures in the foot.

As the disease causes much pain the horse is lame and at rest may point the foot. 'Dry' corns usually respond readily to removal of the cause and a few days' rest, but care should be taken to see that the foot is properly shod afterwards.

The more serious types of corn should have professional attention as they can lead to permanent lameness.

THRUSH – Thrush is usually an avoidable disease. It is an infection in which the tissue around the cleft of the frog becomes soft and discharges a foetid fluid. The commonest cause is standing in liquid manure, and the condition is therefore most often seen in the hind feet of stalled rather than boxed horses. Regular picking out of the feet and cleaning of the standing will prevent trouble.

Mild cases respond to packing the cleft of the frog with a piece of thick string soaked in Stockholm Tar or Tincture of Iodine. Common salt is another useful dressing for this condition. Aerosols as used for foot rot in sheep are useful for treating thrush. Severe cases may need to have the horn trimmed away and the hoof treated under professional guidance.

SIDEBONE – The two sidepieces of the third phalanx are prolonged as the lateral cartilages; these are of rubbery consistence and serve in the circulation of blood in the foot. When pressure is put on the foot by the animal the lateral cartilages bend outwards with each stride. With concussion these cartilages may turn into bone; this does not yield as the cartilage does and the animal may be lame. The ossified cartilages can easily be felt just above the coronary band. In many cases, once they have fully hardened, sidebones cause no further trouble. When they are massive and much larger than the original cartilages they may, however, cause lameness, the treatment for which is surgical removal.

SANDCRACKS – Possibly because they look insignificant in the early stages, sandcracks are often regarded too lightly by horse owners. A sandcrack is a split in the wall of the hoof which extends upwards into the coronary band; it may not always descend to the bottom of the hoof. The cause is probably associated with mineral deficiency or other nutrient failure and the crack occurs when the foot is concussed. The danger is that as the split widens when weight is put on the foot, the sensitive laminae inside the hoof may be trapped in the crack, and become injured and then septic. If this occurs treatment with antibiotics may be necessary.

Sandcracks may be controlled by clipping the edges together or using some contrivance, such as special clips, to attain this end. Surgical shoeing and trimming of the foot to avoid pressure on the wall causing the crack to open, is also needed. If the split damages the coronary band what is termed a 'false quarter' may be caused, and the damaged band will secrete defective horn with a permanent crack. It is desirable in cases of sandcrack that the growth of horn be encouraged by rubbing in cod liver oil. In some cases blistering the coronet or the administration of gelatine is called for.

When the crack reaches the ground surface but does not extend upwards as far as the coronary band it is known as a 'grasscrack' or 'false sandcrack'. Grasscracks can usually be rectified by the farrier, but care should be taken to ensure that they are not made to extend upwards by working without shoes.

SEEDY TOE – This condition seems to be less common than formerly. It is due to the breakdown of the horn at the toe of the foot. The outside of the wall appears normal but when the shoe is removed and the horn pared away it is found that the inner surface of the wall has developed a cavity filled with powdery horn. Tapping the wall elicits a hollow, drumlike sound. Among the causes are tight-fitting shoes, close nails, chronic laminitis, and faulty nutrition. Lameness is rare. Treatment consists of paring away the damaged horn and coating the cavity with Stockholm tar. This treatment will, of course, weaken the wall and special shoeing may be needed to prevent splitting and breaking of the horn.

QUITTOR – A quittor is an abscess which forms in the foot and bursts above the coronary band with a sinus running down close to the horny wall of the hoof. The cause is some infection which has found its way into the hoof. As the pus cannot escape through the horny wall it works upwards and escapes through the skin just above the horn.

Quittor is a serious condition and may put a horse out of

action for a long time, as treatment may necessitate removal of a substantial part of the wall of the hoof if the condition is unresponsive to antibiotic therapy.

PUS IN THE FOOT – Perhaps the commonest of all forms of lameness, pus in the foot has numerous causes. It can follow a prick from a nail during shoeing or a penetrating wound of the sole, as happens when the horse treads on an up-pointing nail when a shoe becomes dislodged. Grit working up can also be responsible.

The affected animal is acutely lame and may hold the foot off the ground. The cause of the trouble should be searched for and removed. Good drainage then has to be provided by paring away the sole, and a poultice applied. With prompt treatment most cases make good recovery.

Wounds in the foot are of the kind that lead to tetanus, and measures must always be taken to ensure that the horse has protection against this infection.

Sometimes a shoe nail is driven 'too close' and the resulting pressure on the sensitive tissues (although they have not been pricked) causes pain and lameness soon after shoeing. This is called 'nail bind' and only needs the offending nail to be withdrawn to correct the condition.

SPAVIN – Spavins are diseases of the hock and are named according to their type; thus there is the bone or 'jack' spavin, the occult spavin, the bog spavin, and the 'blood' spavin. This last is an enlargement of the vein which runs across the front of the hock. The hock is the joint between the tibia above and the cannon bone below, and the joint comprises six bones in two rows (occasionally there are seven bones). These two rows move one against the other as well as against the long bones when the hock is bent. With strain there is inflammation and a bony growth is laid down. When this is visible it is called a 'jack' spavin and is usually seen on the inside of the hock at the top of the cannon bone. If the inflammation occurs between the bones in the centre of the hock it will not be visible and is known as an 'occult' spavin. Such a spavin may, however, be detectable by X-ray.

Spavins are caused by strain, especially by rearing, walking on the hind legs, violent jumping, a sudden increase in pace, or pulling heavy loads in harness.

Often the onset of spavin is gradual. A spavined horse tends to wear the shoe at the toe. Spavin is a 'warming out' lameness, and often the lameness disappears after a few minutes' work. If the leg is held with the hock flexed for a minute or so ('jack-knifing the hock') there may be a marked increase in lameness when the horse is made to trot immediately; this test should not, however, be regarded as infallible.

If care is taken not to strain the hock further – if it is given complete rest – a spavin will often consolidate adjoining bones and the horse will recover full usefulness, albeit with perhaps a slight loss of flexion in the hock. In other cases firing, blistering or corticosteroids are called for. Of first importance, however, is complete rest and if this precaution is neglected, what might have been only a temporary lameness can endanger the future usefulness of the animal. Surgical treatment to fix the bones of the hock together is sometimes needed.

BOG SPAVIN – This is a soft enlargement of the hock due to excess fluid in the hock joint. It resembles an articular windgall, but the swelling appears in three places: in front of the hock towards the inside, and smaller swellings on each side at the back of the joint. Bog spavin is a blemish but rarely causes trouble. Such treatments as are effective are quite complicated and seldom necessary.

THOROUGHPIN – So-called because someone thought it resembled a pin that could be pushed through from one side of the hock to the other, although 'thoroughpeg' would be more descriptive, a thoroughpin is a swelling of the synovial sheath above the hock. There is an increase in the amount of fluid, forming a swelling on either the inside or the outside of the hock towards the rear. When pressure is put on the swelling it disappears and a similar swelling comes on the other side of the hock.

The cause is strain and there is usually no lameness or apparent discomfort. Often the swelling will decrease if the horse is rested but in other cases the enlargement is chronic. Because it is no more than an eyesore many owners are content to leave a thoroughpin alone; however, mild blistering often induces a thickening in the overlying skin which compresses the swelling and reduces it, and tight bandaging with cotton wool providing pressure may have the same effect. When circumstances justify it the surgical aspiration of the fluid and its partial replacement by corticosteroids is frequently successful.

SPRAINED HOCK – This is comparable with sprained ankle in man, and is just as painful. Often it is the precursor of bone spavin and it has similar causes. Treatment comprises complete rest and the prevention of excessive inflammation by cold douches and cold water bandages. Over-anxiety to return the horse to work is likely to lead to bone deposition and the formation of spavin.

CAPPED HOCK – This unsightly swelling appears on the point of the hock as a result of injury, perhaps due to kicking in the stable. It is an increase in the fluid content of the bursa (synovial sac) under the tendon and, like other similar swellings, often causes trouble by its unsightliness. Lameness is seldom present, but the blemish is usually permanent. Again, early cold applications may prevent an increase in size. The skin over the swelling thickens with time and an enlargement persists even if the fluid is removed. Blisters help to reduce the unsightliness, but by altering the lie of the hair or its colour may draw attention to the condition. Again, surgical aspiration of the fluid and associated treatment may help.

STRINGHALT – This is a nervous affliction of one or both hind legs, characterized by a peculiarity of gait in which the affected limb is snatched up higher than normal, sometimes almost kicking the belly. The condition comes and goes at first but tends to persist longer as it progresses. Often the peculiarity is more marked if the horse is backed and turned. Highwaymen of old were said to treat the condition by massive firing with the blade of a red-hot shovel, but the law-abiding horse owner may prefer to

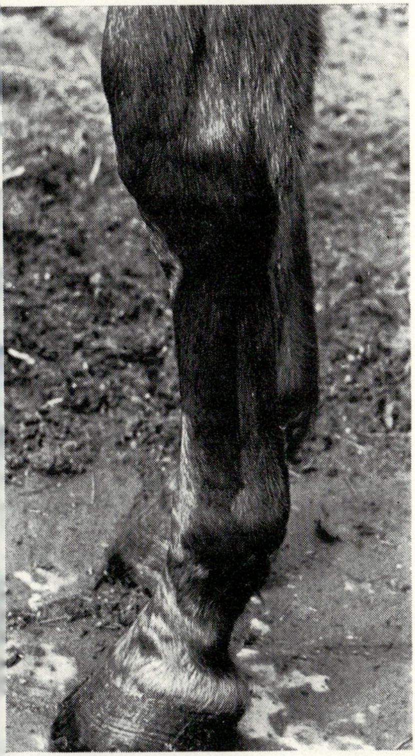

1. Bumped knee: large soft swelling in front and above the knee of a show jumper.

2. Splint: inside the right foreleg.

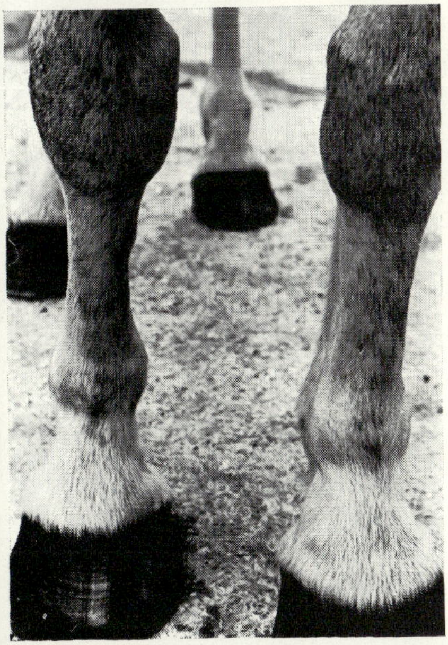

3. Capped elbow.

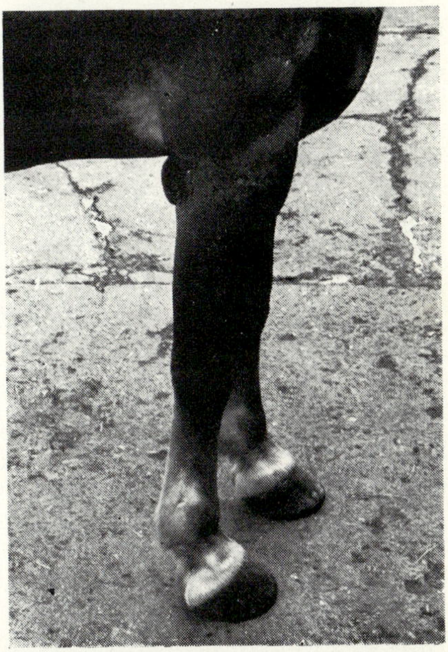

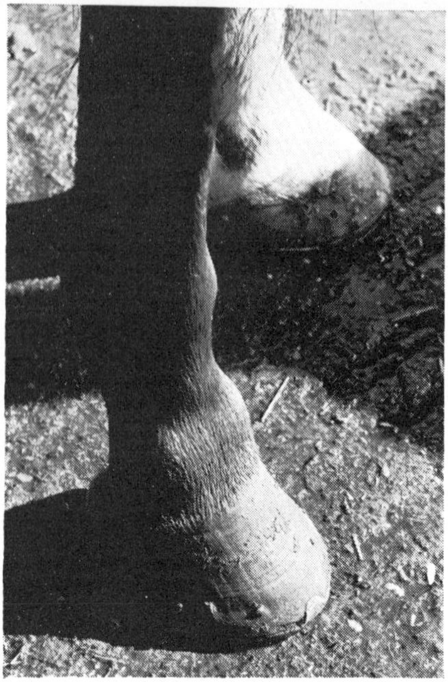

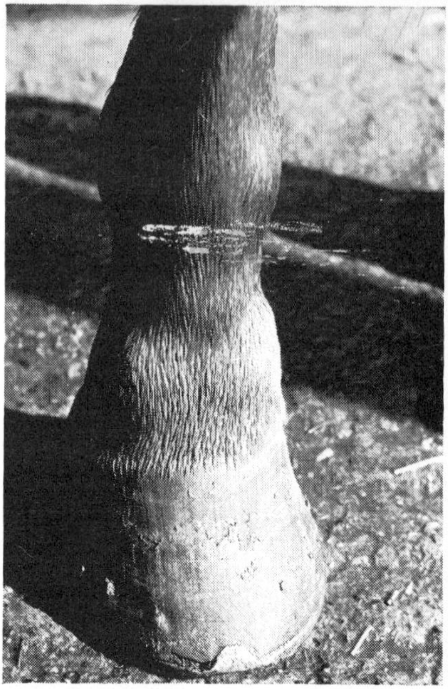

4 & 5. Ringbone.

6. Sandcrack: a typical sandcrack causing lameness in the left forefoot.

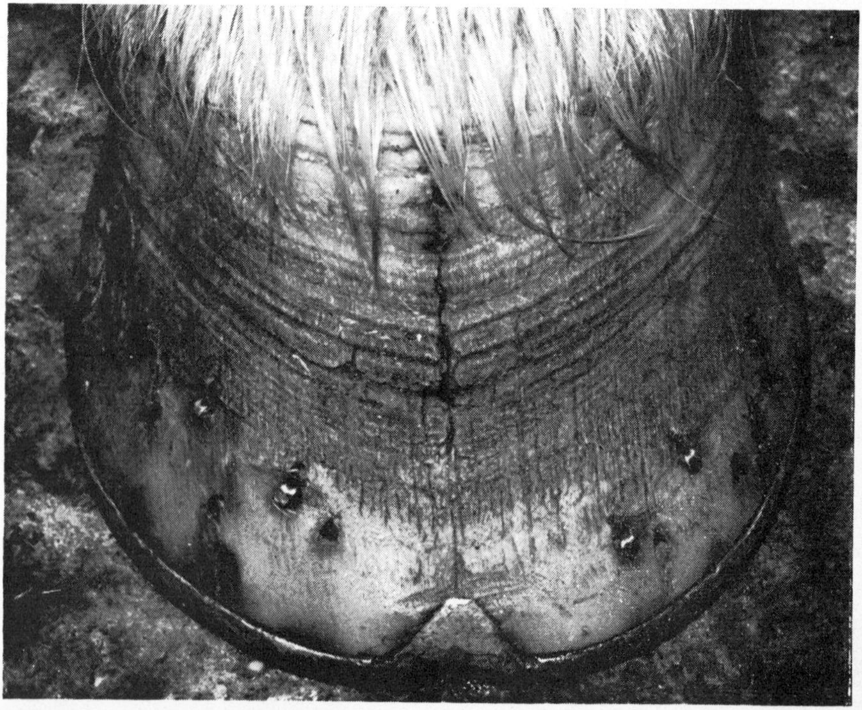

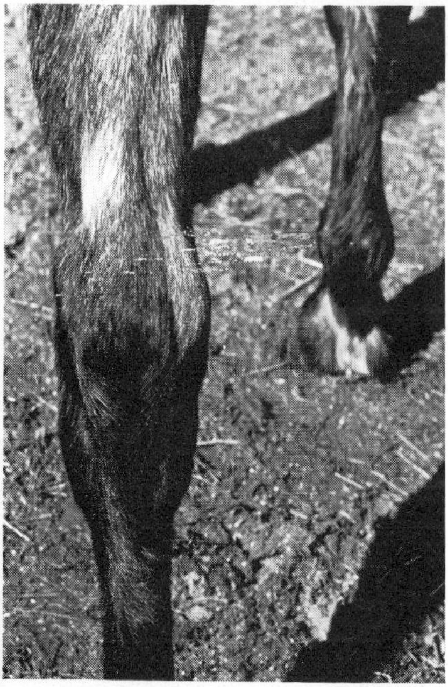
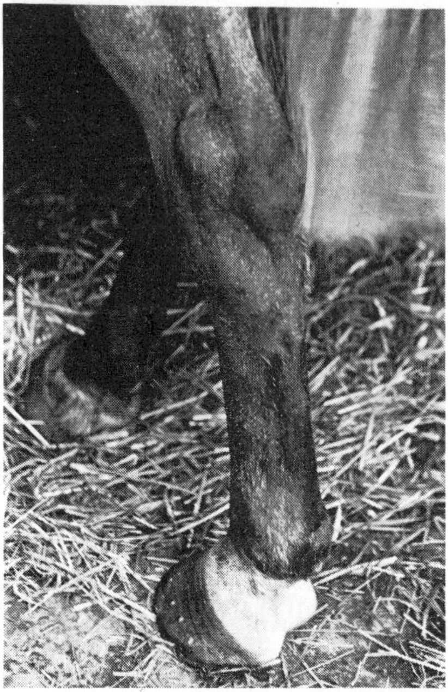

7–10. Thoroughpin: these photographs show the positions into which the thoroughpin can move.

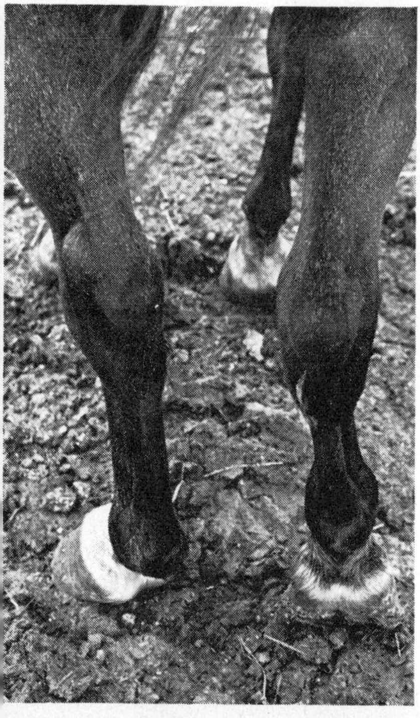
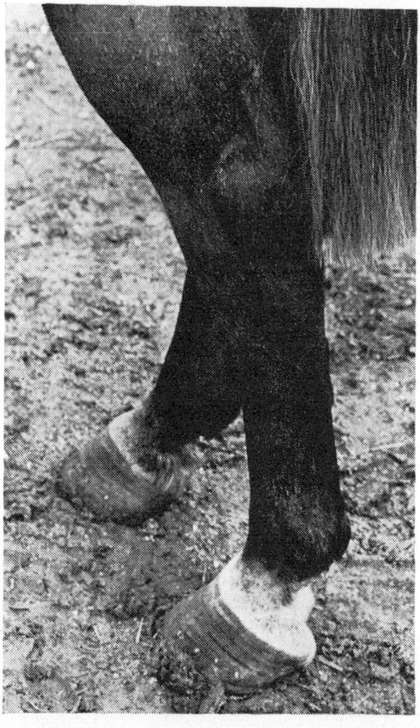

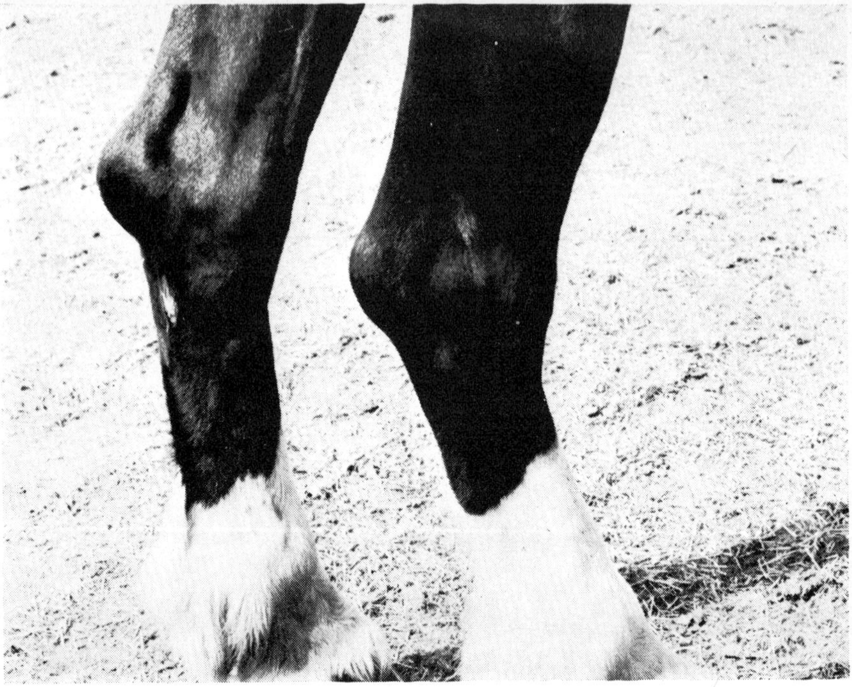

11. Capped hock.

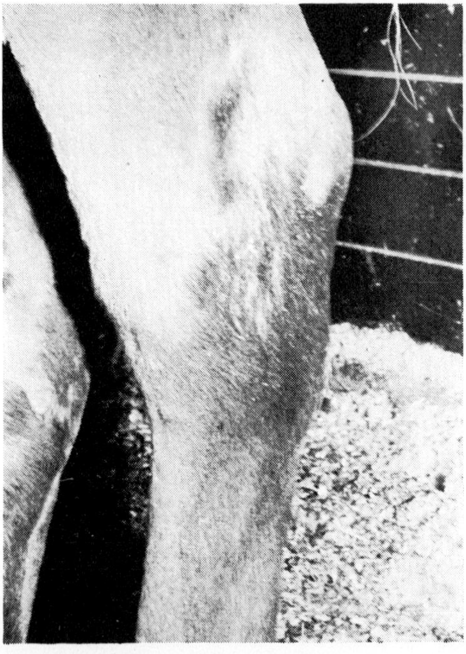

12. Curb.

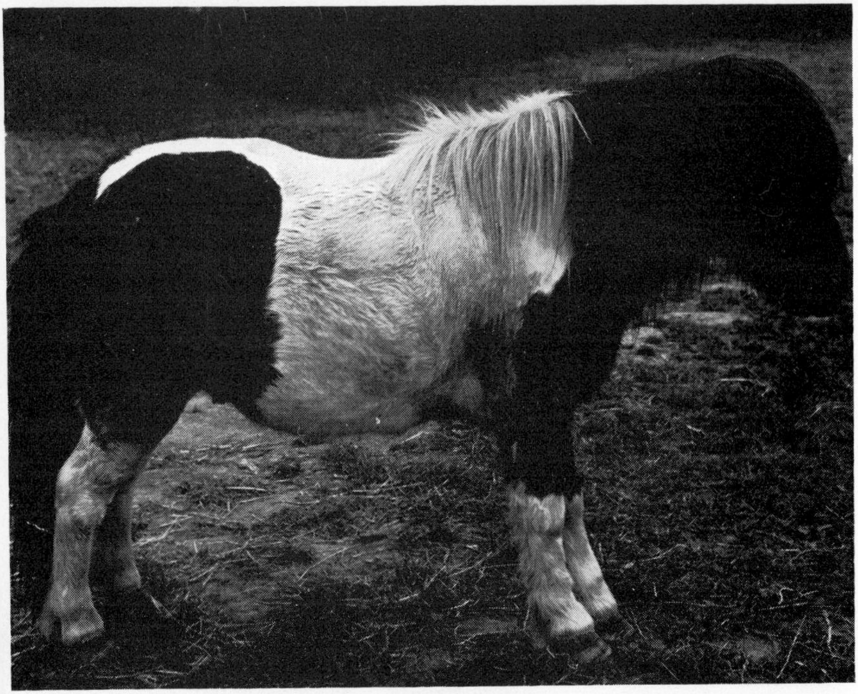

13. Laminitis: note the typical stance with forefeet advanced and weight on the heels.

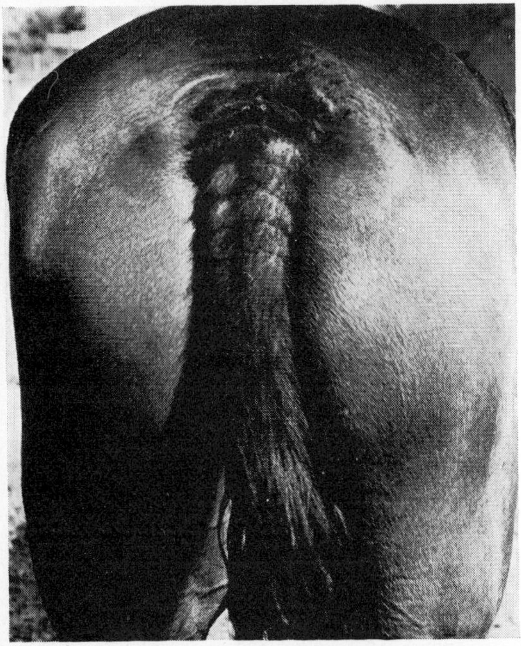

14. Sweet itch.

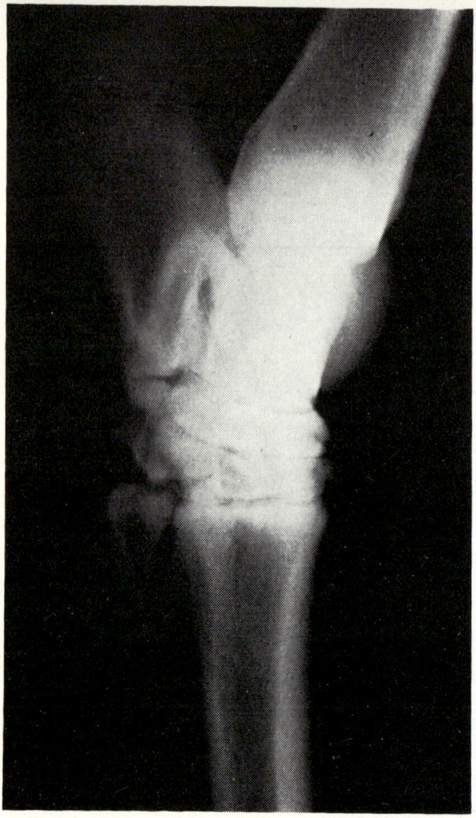

15 & 16. X-rays of hock from side and front showing the rows of bones and spaces between them.

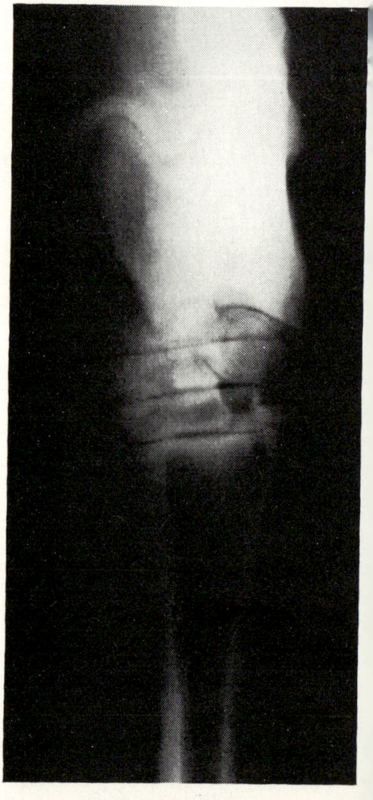

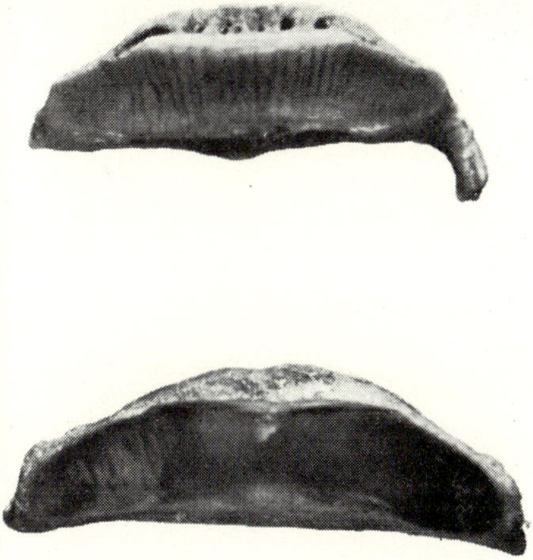

17. Navicular disease: normal navicular bone below, navicular bone with osteophyte above.

8. Spavin: bones from a spavined hock howing the layers of bones fused with the op of the cannon bone.

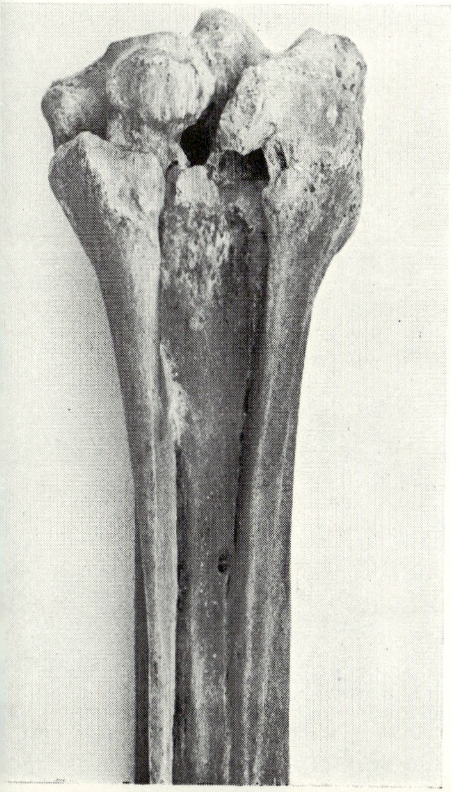

19. Splint: fore cannon bone with splint.

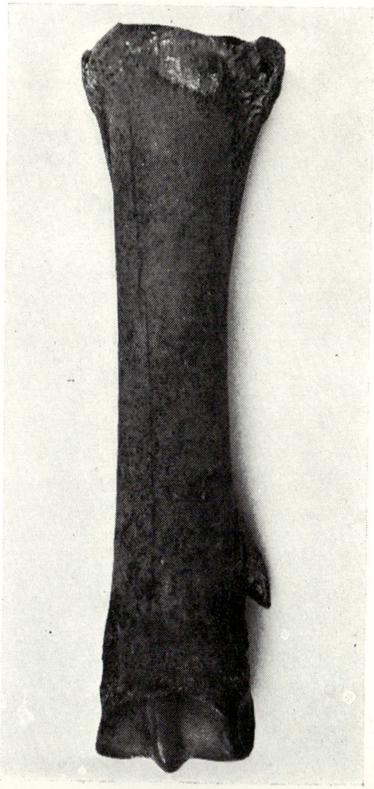

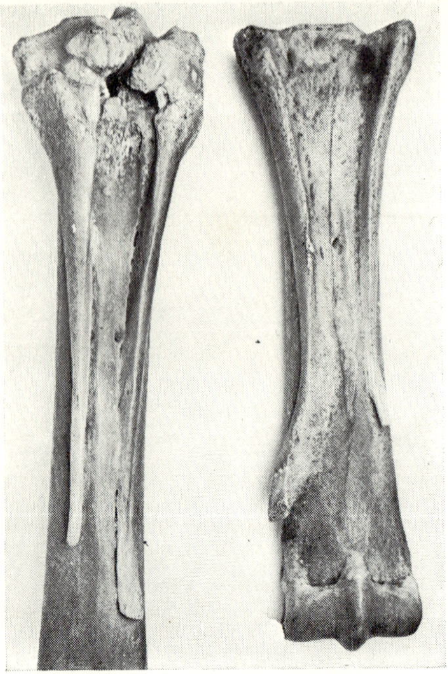

20. Spavin and splint: hind cannon bone with spavin, and fore cannon bone with splint, both from the same horse.

21. Ringbone: normal phalanges.

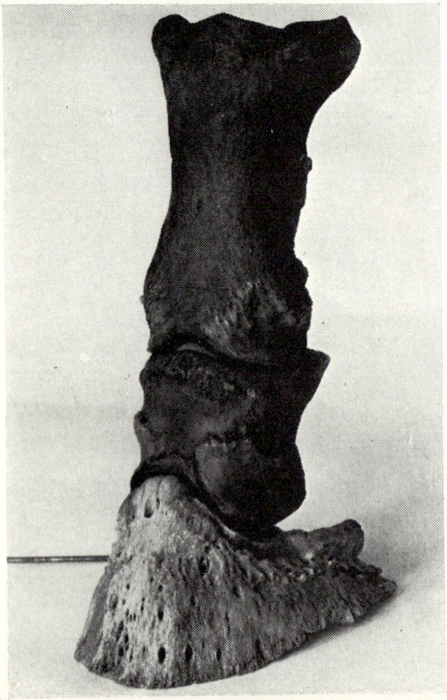

22. Ringbone.

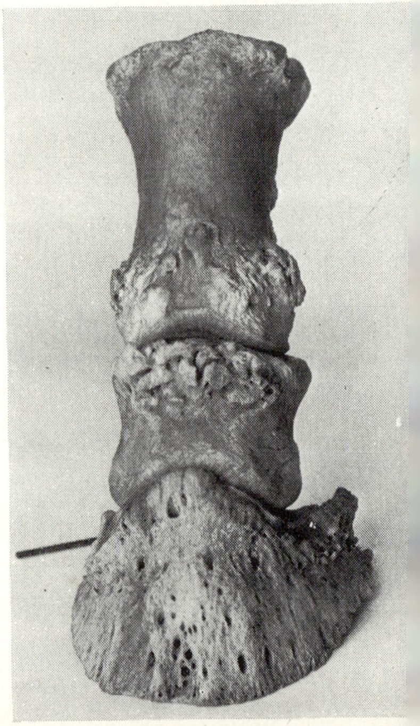

consult his veterinary surgeon, who might advise cutting one of the tendons near the hock or, conservatively, point out that many affected horses continue to work usefully for years without treatment.

DISLOCATED PATELLA – The patella or knee cap lies to the front of the stifle joint and is attached to the powerful muscles above, transmitting their pull to the bones below the stifle. Sometimes the patella slips out of the groove in the femur in which it normally runs and the horse is unable to bend the leg. While it sometimes goes back of its own accord, more often it has to be replaced by a veterinary sugeon. This condition is commonest in ponies in poor condition and may call for surgical treatment.

CURBS – A curb is a sprain of the ligament at the back of the hock which unites the bone forming the point of the hock with the cannon bone. Excessive contraction by the muscles which attach to the point of the hock will cause this sprain; such contraction occurs when a horse takes much strain on the hocks, as in rearing or jumping at slow paces. The condition is detected by an outward bowing of the line at the back of the cannon to the point of the hock. This is more readily detectable if the hairs are laid by wetting and smoothing with a brush. The affected animal is in pain and lame on the affected leg or legs (often both are sprained). Treatment consists of rest and cold applications. Counter-irritation with liniments, blisters or firing is sometimes used in chronic cases, but rest is usually the best treatment. To avoid blemishing show horses' curbs are often treated with a mild blister, the slight remaining thickening being removed by rubbing in iodine ointment or Scott's dressing, followed by stroking with a toothbrush handle or deer bone (as is used for boning boots) daily for a month or so. Weak, 'sickle' hocks are the most liable to this form of sprain and are therefore sometimes called 'curby hocks' even before the tell-tale bowing occurs. Most cases of curb make complete recovery to usefulness.

Chapter 4

THE ALIMENTARY SYSTEM

The importance of the alimentary system being in good order for the maintenance of health needs no emphasis.

TEETH – The horse uses its incisor or cutting teeth to graze grass, bite mouthfuls from a net of hay and so on. The food in the mouth is then chewed between the molar teeth or grinders and mixed with saliva before being formed into a bolus and swallowed.

Defects of conformation, as when the upper jaw is too long or too short, or when the molars form a wavy line with their grinding surfaces, do not always cause trouble. An extreme form of over-shot upper jaw (parrot mouth) may cause difficulty in grazing so that the animal loses condition when at grass. However, if an adult animal is not suffering from lack of flesh it has obviously been able to cope with this defect.

Tartared teeth are coated with a hard, brittle deposit; the condition is unsightly and may cause offensive breath. Large deposits on the tushes may result in inflammation of the gums or, in extreme cases, even interfere with the bit.

It can be cracked and scraped from the teeth with forceps and scalers.

Wolf teeth are small teeth which grow in front of the large molars and are usually not present, although they are considered part of the normal dentition of the horse. In the past they have been blamed for many things including lameness and vice. They may cause trouble in bitting and some head shakers behave normally when these teeth have been removed. Their removal is not, of course, a job for the amateur owner.

Because the upper jaw of the horse is wider than the lower, in the normal course of wear the upper molars are worn away on the tongue side and the lower ones on the cheek side so that a sharp edge develops on the outer side of the upper molars and on the inner side of the lower ones. These edges are in some cases very sharp indeed and one can sustain a severely cut finger by feeling them. Not surprisingly, these sharp edges can cut the horse's cheeks or tongue and so cause pain. The pain makes the horse liable to bolt its food without thorough mastication and, if the animal is fed on hard food, grains of whole oats and the like may pass through and be seen in the droppings. Faulty mastication leads to poor digestion with consequent loss of condition or even colic. The horse may drop food out of its mouth while chewing – this is called 'quidding'. The sharp edges on these teeth can be taken off with a special rasp. Broken teeth may also have sharp edges and these, too, can be filed smooth.

Gingivitis, or inflammation of the gums, occurs most commonly in young horses when they are teething. When the teeth have fully erupted the condition disappears. The discomfort may be enough to put the horse off its feed or to make him resent the bit. Tincture of myrrh is the established remedy for this and should be painted on the inflamed gums several times a day.

LAMPAS – this term denotes swelling of the mucous membrane covering the hard palate behind the incisor teeth. When feeding this swells and the ridges become more prominent, enabling the horse to retain food in its mouth. During teething and when the mouth is sore the swelling sometimes persists. If it is excessive four tablespoonfuls of Epsom salts in the drinking water for a few days is generally enough to put things right. At one time barbarous treatments such as lancing or burning the palate were advocated, but such cruel practices are needless.

TONGUE INJURIES – injuries to the tongue may be due to bits which are of the wrong size, worn, or badly made, but they are most often caused by roughness and bad hands or by the misuse of tongue straps or bootlaces and the like used to tie down the tongue. Treatment consists of removing, and preferably not re-introducing, the cause. The horse must be exercised with a bitless bridle, or in hand on a headcollar, until the wounds have healed. A dilute solution of permanganate of potash (enough to colour the solution pink) makes a good mouthwash to use after feeding.

CHOKE – When the horse has masticated its mouthful of food and has mixed it with saliva it swallows the bolus. Usually this passes straight down the oesophagus or gullet into the stomach, but occasionally it becomes stuck on the way down and causes choking. This seems to appear most often in animals in poor condition, and among the more frequent causes are the feeding of sugar beet pulp which has not been sufficiently soaked before feeding. A bolus of sugar beet pulp grows in size as it absorbs saliva, and carrots or similar root vegetables when cut into discs and swallowed without chewing can also become stuck in the gullet. Bolting dry grain, too, is an oft-reported cause. The condition is alarming and the horse shows signs of distress and makes gulping movements. Saliva mixed with food comes down the nostrils and out of the mouth. If the obstruction can be felt in the neck it is sometimes possible to shift it upwards towards the mouth by pressing with the fingers. When the obstruction is in the pharynx, or back of the mouth, one may be able to draw the tongue out of the mouth with one hand and remove the obstruction with the other. There should be no need to mention that unless he is careful the operator runs considerable risk of being severely bitten. Most obstructions, unfortunately, occur in that part of the gullet running through the chest.

More severe cases need the attention of a veterinary surgeon who may use drugs to relax the muscle of the oesophagus and lubricate the bolus on its way down, or may employ special instruments to push the mass onwards into the stomach or to pull it upwards into the mouth. In other cases he will use a stomach tube to wash away the obstruction bit by bit, or even two tubes – one up each nostril – pumping fluid into one and letting it run out through the other.

BOT INFESTATION – The horse bot fly lays eggs in the autumn on the hairs of horses' legs. When the horse licks its limbs these eggs stuck on the hairs are stimulated to hatch by moisture, warmth and friction, and tiny maggots enter the horse's mouth. These burrow under the covering of the tongue and mouth and later grow and are swallowed into the stomach. When in the mouth they cause slight irritation and are one cause of 'laughing horses', photographs of which showing the animals with open mouths and bared teeth are so often seen in the popular press.

In the stomach the maggots grow to about $\frac{3}{4}$ in. long and $\frac{1}{4}$ in. in diameter, and one end burrows into the wall of the stomach. At post-mortem examinations stomachs are often found to contain masses of these grubs covering half or more of the stomach wall. Although they have been known to rupture the stomach it is seldom that they cause the host any harm other than possible indigestion. At a later stage of the development of the parasite, the bots will be found in the dung.

Infested horses can be treated with a variety of drugs, some of which, such as carbon tetrachloride, are dangerous if improperly used. Prevention is better than cure and the eggs should be removed daily from the legs of horses. No fluids are very good for this, although rubbing with a paraffin-soaked rag, or the use of a neat household detergent washed off with warm water after a few minutes, have been recommended. It is quickest, generally, to scrape the eggs off the hairs with a knife or safety razor.

WORMS – Horses are hosts to tapeworms and round worms. Tapeworms are not a very common problem, and can sometimes be eradicated by the administration of half an ounce of freshly ground areca nut – or your veterinary surgeon will supply you with a medicament.

Ascarids are the most frightening round worms in appearance to the owner. They are white or yellowish in colour, $\frac{1}{4}$ in. in diameter and as much as a foot long. After successful medication a horse may evacuate a gallon of such worms. These worms will respond to treatment which your veterinary surgeon will supply.

But the really dangerous worms are the red worms, or Strongyles. These little worms, $\frac{1}{4}$ in. to $1\frac{1}{2}$ in. long, are of several species, and are responsible for the death and unthriftiness of a large proportion of our equine population. The horse becomes infested with these worms from the pastures which are said to be 'horse sick' when there has been a build-up of infestation over the years. Quite young foals can become infected when turned out and the infective form of the worms will persist on hay made from infested pastures. Foalhood infestation may lead to colic in adult life.

Pastures can be rendered safer by regular dosing of horses grazing on them, by grazing with non-susceptible animals such as sheep, in rotation with horses, and by picking up the droppings daily and putting them on a manure heap whose heat will destroy the worms as they develop. Harrowing the field regularly so as to spread out the dung and dry it will keep down the infestation.

When the infective form of the worm has been swallowed it enters the stomach and intestines of the horse and then burrows right through into the abdominal cavity. The larvae at this stage may enter one of the main blood vessels to the bowel and develop in its wall, producing what is known as a verminous aneurism. This may take months to develop but eventually so interferes with the blood supply to the bowel that the animal suffers from indigestion, colic or enteritis and fails to thrive or becomes under-nourished and dies. Other worm larvae travel to practically all parts of the body, but eventually find their way back to the intestine where they burrow into the lining and suck blood. This results in anaemia and interferes with the absorption of nourishment, leading to a thin, unthrifty animal. Death may occur in severe cases.

The presence of the worms can be determined by laboratory examination of the droppings. This will show both the parasites and the eggs in the faeces.

There are numerous effective proprietary medicines for red worms, but it is important that preventive measures much as those outlined above should be taken as well as using medicine.

The oxyuris worm lives in the large intestine and the female worm lays its eggs around the horse's anus. These eggs can be seen as cream-coloured waxy masses. The worms cause irritation and infested animals rub their tails and lose condition because of restlessness. There are several proprietary drugs effective against the worms. Carbolic ointment will kill the eggs and allay the itching. Thorough cleaning of the stable is indicated.

COLIC – Colic is a term applied to pain in the abdomen. There are many causes but by far the most frequent is indigestion. Failure to digest the food properly also arises from many causes, including sudden changes of diet, irregular feeding times, poor quality of food, over-feeding a tired horse, exercising too soon after eating, the feeding of sweets (sometimes with the wrappers still on!), green apples, sandwiches and the like, which frequently occurs when horses are kept in a field to which the public have access.

The symptoms of colic are restlessness, pawing at the ground, looking round at the belly, sweating (sometimes in patches), groaning, lying down and rising, rolling, cold ears and a dejected look. In those cases where there is impaction of the bowels scanty faeces or no faeces at all will be passed; diarrhoea may indicate that there is inflammation of the bowels.

'Spasmodic' colic is the commonest type. The pain comes and goes and the animal appears at ease between attacks. When the bowel is thrown into a spasm it causes pain and this may lead to further spasms so that the condition is progressive. If one can relieve the pain early in the attack it is often possible to prevent further spasms. The administration of pain-relieving drugs is therefore called for. As some cases do not respond to first aid, professional treatment may be needed and it is wise to have by you colic drinks supplied by your own veterinary surgeon, so that if he has to be summoned his subsequent treatment is facilitated. Proprietary drenches, although often good, may contain substances which contra-indicate certain types of after-treatment.

In addition to giving pain relievers, keep the horse warm with clothing. If it sweats, rub the animal dry. Opinions differ with regard to letting the horse roll. It seems to relieve the pain and therefore should be permitted on humane grounds, but there is a school of thought which believes that rolling is liable to induce twist of the gut which in many cases has a fatal result. Whether rolling is a result or cause of twist, rolling in the confined space of an unpadded stable may injure the horse or cause it to be cast by getting its feet under a manger or other fixture. Probably the best procedure is to keep the horse quietly on the move by leading it around the stable yard. Do not be tempted to lead it too far away from the stable lest it lie down in an inconvenient place and refuse to rise.

The application of warmth to the abdomen with hot water bottles gives comfort.

A warning should be given that a horse lying down or rolling with colic is apt to kick without warning and attendants should be circumspect in their movements to avoid the risk of being kicked. It is always as well to put on a headcollar in the early stages of a bout of colic so that some measure of control can be maintained throughout the attack.

When the colic is due to some irritant in the bowel, such as unripe apples, the attack will usually be self-limiting as the purging which takes place eliminates the irritant substance. A purgative such as Epsom salts in a dose of 6 oz. in half a gallon of water will hasten things along, but a warning must be given that the use of such substances when the diagnosis is mistaken may not only lengthen the period of illness, but also cause the patient additional suffering. If first aid does not give prompt relief do not delay sending for professional assistance, lest a curable case develops into a fatal one.

Whatever the cause of an attack of colic, treatment should be aimed at keeping the horse out of pain and preventing it from injuring itself. An Australian veterinary surgeon once wrote that before treating a case of colic he always prayed that nothing he did would cause the horse to have more pain than it had to begin with.

Chapter 5

THE RESPIRATORY SYSTEM

The respiratory system includes the nasal passages, larynx, windpipe, lungs and diaphragm. In the horse the respiratory system is subject to many diseases, and as the animal has by the nature of things to do hard and fast work these diseases are of great importance.

NASAL CATARRH – In popular usage catarrh means the discharge from one or both nostrils of a thick, creamy discharge often coloured green or yellow and sometimes with an offensive odour (when it is called *ozena*). The cause of the condition is inflammation of the mucous membranes which line the upper respiratory passages. Commonly, the discharge comes from both nostrils and is due to inflammation of the mucous membrane of the turbinate bones over which inspired air flows. Apart from snorting to remove the mucus the horse may show no other signs of being unwell, but in more severe cases there will be a loss of appetite and a rise in temperature and sometimes there is a cough. It is not unusual for blood to appear in the discharge.

Simple cases respond to steam inhalations which render

the discharges thinner and by clearing the nasal passages make breathing easier and the patient more comfortable. The nose should be cleaned daily with warm boracic solution or other mild antiseptic and the area likely to be affected by discharge covered with petroleum jelly to prevent soreness.

Drainage is encouraged by turning any animal with a nasal discharge out to grass, and this is beneficial in most cases.

Cases of catarrh which do not respond to simple treatment may need thorough investigation before a diagnosis can be made and proper treatment given. When only one nostril is involved the cause may be in the sinuses (air spaces) in the bones of the skull, perhaps because of infection of a tooth root. The horse possesses two sacs in its head, known as guttural pouches, and inflammation of these may also result in a nasal discharge, usually seen when the head is lowered. Simple treatments are often of no avail here and treatment or even diagnosis may necessitate the use of general anaesthesia.

PNEUMONIA – Pneumonia is not a common ailment of the horse and when it does occur it is usually in very young, old or debilitated animals. Such inflammation of the lungs may follow what appears to be nasal catarrh, or it may complicate an infectious disease such as strangles. Affected horses are obviously ill and have high temperatures and difficulty in breathing. The condition is serious and unless promptly and properly treated may end in death. Make the horse as comfortable as you can in well-ventilated, draught-free quarters and send for assistance.

COUGH – Coughing is a symptom of disease rather than a disease itself. It is caused by irritation of the sensitive covering of the air passages. When these coverings are healthy then gross irritation, as by the inhalation of dust, will cause a reflex cough in an endeavour to expel the offending foreign matter. When the irritant is persistent then the animal produces more mucus whose object is to entrap the irritant material. A cough will then drive the mucus and entrapped irritant towards the mouth. The trachea, or windpipe, is lined with cells bearing microscopic hairs pointing towards the mouth; as the mucus is driven upwards by the cough these hairs prevent it slipping down again so that eventually it can be expelled as sputum. That is what happens in the healthy animal, but when the irritant is constantly applied (as when dusty hay is fed) the cells become excessively sensitive and the horse will cough with little or no cause, or it may be that the cells continue to produce mucus when the irritant is no longer being applied to them and the horse will cough to rid itself of the unnecessary phlegm.

There are numerous specific diseases which inflame the respiratory passages and produce coughing as a symptom. These diseases include epidemic cough, influenza, strangles, and broken wind, which are described in later paragraphs.

A simple cough should be treated by removing the cause of the irritation (e.g. dusty hay); and it is a wise precaution to damp such hay as is given so that any dust shall be rendered less irritating. Both clover hay and dusty bedding tend to aggravate coughs.

When there has been an acute inflammation of the air

passages a residual hyper-sensitivity may persist in an apparently recovered horse and cause coughing in response to a very mild stimulus. Thus horses may cough when first taken out of their stables on a cold day or when first moved into a faster pace which causes deeper breathing, the inhalation of cold air then being enough to irritate the passages and cause coughing which, however, disappears when the animal warms up.

Simple cough may be successfully treated with proprietary cough electuaries or linctuses, but when it persists or other symptoms are shown the owner is justified in calling in professional advice.

Many coughs are associated with stable ventilation and disappear when plenty of fresh air is provided by leaving the stable door open day and night. Of course this may take some of the shine off the horse's coat and, in any case, adequate clothing must be provided. On the other hand there are a few cases, very few, in which the reverse is true and coughing only stops when the stable is kept warm at the expense of adequate ventilation: but it must be emphasized that these are a very small minority.

The administration of four tablespoonfuls of cod liver oil daily in the food is of benefit both in treatment and prevention of cough.

ROARING AND WHISTLING – When a horse breathes air into its lungs the air passes between the vocal cords in the larynx at the top of the trachea. In horses (the condition is rare in ponies) it is not uncommon for the nerves of one (nearly always the left) or both of these cords to become paralysed so that the cords are not drawn out of the way of the air stream. This results in insufficient air reaching the lungs with impairment of the animal's efficiency. The offending cord vibrates in the flow of air and makes a noise during respiration. This may be high pitched (whistling) or lower (roaring) and animals which make such inspiratory sounds are regarded as unsound. The noise is not heard all the time even in an affected animal and it may sometimes be accentuated by riding the horse in a circle with maximum flexion. In other cases the sound is only heard when the horse is galloped hard for a long distance.

In many cases roaring is a sequel to strangles or other infectious diseases, and numerous cases have been caused by poisoning from lead or certain plants.

Although a slight degree of this condition may not seriously interfere with an animal doing only light work, palliative measures should be taken to try to avoid the condition getting worse. Rest is essential. Dusty food and environment should be avoided and the stable must be well-ventilated. More serious cases can only be dealt with by surgical removal of the cords under anaesthesia or by the insertion of a tube (tubing) into the trachea below the larynx so that the inspired air does not pass between the vocal cords. The advisability of either of these courses of action is a matter to be discussed with a veterinary surgeon.

Roaring and whistling should not be confused with 'high blowing' which is a noise made in the nostrils of healthy horses when they are breathing out at fast paces.

BROKEN WIND – The anatomy of the lungs has been likened to a bunch of grapes. The windpipe (trachea) divides into the bronchi, which divide again and again into smaller and smaller bronchioles, the smallest of which end in a minute sac. This sac is very thin walled and has a copious blood supply. Oxygen from the air inside the sac passes through the thin wall into the blood, and carbon dioxide from the blood passes in the reverse direction and is eliminated with the expired air. Under certain circumstances the walls of these sacs, or alveoli as they are called, burst so that instead of one bronchiole bringing air to one small sac, several bronchioles supply one larger cavity. Just as if, when the interior walls of a many-roomed house are knocked down then less wall paper is required, so when these alveoli are ruptured there is less area in contact with the blood and gaseous exchange is reduced. This is the condition known as pulmonary emphysema, broken wind, or heaves.

Broken wind is a disease of older horses and the symptoms are a chronic wheezy cough, often persisting throughout the night. The animal tires easily. As the condition worsens there is more difficulty with breathing, the animal is unable to extract the normal amount of oxygen from a given volume of inspired air and therefore has to take in more air in a given time. In addition, the elasticity of the small alveoli having been lost, the air is not automatically expelled from the lungs and the animal has to make an extra effort to express the last of the air from its lungs. This effort shows by a double expiratory movement which is easily seen on watching the flank. The curve of the last ribs also shows more prominently than usual.

The causes of the condition are not fully understood,

but some horses may show signs of the disease when working in certain districts and appear free from symptoms when moved elsewhere. Swiss and Swedish workers find that there are more cases of broken wind in those years when the hay crop is bad. They suggest that a fungus makes the hay mouldy and causes an asthmatic type of condition.

Any severe bout of coughing is liable to extend the disease by rupturing further alveoli.

There is no hope of a cure when the disease exists and treatment is aimed at preventing any worsening of the condition. Caught early the animal may retain much of its usefulness.

The rules for the management of a broken-winded horse are:

1. Never feed dusty hay, and avoid clover hay.

2. Feed Timothy hay. It is said that the use of gorse hay, made by cutting gorse when not in flower, chaffing it and feeding two double handfuls daily mixed with other non-dusty chaff, will give relief and prevent aggravation of the condition.

3. Feed small feeds and often.

4. Allow at least an hour, preferably more, to elapse after eating any food (even grass) before the horse is worked. The reason for this is that the stomach lies against the diaphragm and if the stomach is full it hinders the free movement of the diaphragm and makes breathing even more difficult.

5. Administer daily doses of cod liver oil.

6. Give as much fresh air as possible.

7. Use peat moss or sawdust as bedding, as they do not contain irritating substances.

STRANGLES – Although this is a systemic disease the respiratory symptoms are the most prominent. It is an infectious and contagious disease of horses, mainly affecting young ones. Like measles in humans, most youngsters get it, recover and are immune for the rest of their lives.

Horses usually first come in contact with the disease when they leave home and travel on public transport or go into dealers' yards, and it is 4–10 days later that symptoms are first seen. In America it is called 'shipping fever'. Affected animals lose their appetites, are depressed and have a high temperature (104–106°F.) They develop a nasal discharge and the lymph glands under the jaw enlarge and become tender. Later these form abscesses and burst with the release of large quantities of pus. There is often a cough which may persist for several weeks.

Prevention consists of avoiding contact with cases of the disease, either direct or indirect, because it can be spread by contaminated grooming kit, feeding or watering utensils, or horse boxes. Vaccines and sera are available through professional channels.

When a horse develops the disease it should be taken off work and isolated under warm conditions. If there is a nasal discharge steaming will help. Abscesses in the lymph glands should be fomented with applications of hot antiseptic solutions and any contaminated material should be burned. Nasal discharges should be bathed away with antiseptic and the nostrils smeared with petroleum jelly or other bland ointment to prevent erosion. A low diet of hay and bran mashes is indicated.

In some cases antibiotics, such as penicillin or oxy-tetracycline or the sulpha drugs, are called for.

Strangles abscesses can develop in other parts of the body ('bastard strangles') and have fatal results. A continuous high temperature usually points to internal abscess formation.

When the abscesses are fomented they will usually burst spontaneously and discharge their contents, with an improvement in the condition of the patient. In other cases the abscesses 'point' and must be lanced.

INFLUENZA – Although infection from man is not a major danger the horse is susceptible to certain of the influenza viruses and in recent years there have been extensive outbreaks of influenza in Great Britain resulting in the cancellation of race meetings, hunting and show jumping, and other sporting events.

The main symptoms are malaise and cough. The cough is often deep and harsh and while it may only be heard once or twice a day the coughing spell may last several minutes. There is not always a high temperature.

Isolation is important and in the event of an outbreak in a district horse owners are advised to avoid contact with other horses. This may lead to a revival of that delightful pastime: solitary, non-competitive horsemanship.

Like the common cold in man, the disease has to run its course but complications may need special treatment. Such complications are best avoided by absolute rest, a light diet and the easing of the cough by electuaries or linctuses. Exercise will aggravate the disease and prolong its course.

An effective preventive vaccine is available but stocks are apt to run out in times of outbreaks and it is wise to have one's horse regularly vaccinated so that it already has resistance should an epidemic occur.

The disease so seriously interferes with racing that an International Veterinary Committee on Equine Influenza has been set up by the Jockey Clubs of Great Britain, Ireland and France. The Committee has recommended that all racehorses be vaccinated, but it points out that such vaccination only protects against currently known influenza viruses, and that there are several other viruses which may cause coughing in horses.

EPIDEMIC COUGH – This is an infectious and contagious condition which spreads rapidly through a stable. Palliative measures should be applied and professional advice sought.

Chapter 6

THE SKIN

Dermatitis is a general term for inflammation of the skin or derma. All skin conditions involving inflammation are therefore properly called dermatitis, but when the specific cause is known, as in *mange*, then it usually has a special name. If the condition of the skin is abnormal but there is no inflammation then the condition is called *dermatosis*. Thus all skin diseases come under the heading of dermatosis, and dermatitis covers those with inflammation. It is essential to try to find out the cause of the disease before starting treatment. However, cleanliness will benefit all diseased conditions and mild antiseptic treatment (in which the antiseptic is sufficiently dilute not to irritate the skin) will help in some cases and be harmful in few or none.

SWEET ITCH – This is an exudative condition usually affecting the mane and tail – parts which have a covering of coarse, thick hair. It is usually seen in the late spring, summer and autumn. The condition causes intense itching and the affected animal rubs the part to such an extent that severe damage may be done by its attempts to relieve the irritation.

The cause of sweet itch is not yet known for certain, but it may be an allergy to certain foods. Good results have been claimed for benzyl benzoate, a chemical whose therapeutic action is dependent upon its parasiticidal qualities. Other people claim success following the application of sulphonamide; however, as this drug is bactericidal in effect and no bacteria have been associated with the condition it is likely that any good effect it may have is associated with its action in drying up the secretions plus, perhaps, the fact that the dried crusts are being removed. Some advocate stabling horses by day and turning out at night, thus avoiding irritation by insects especially gnats. Recently beneficent effects have been claimed for the administration of thyroid extract in small doses. The disease is often treated by veterinary surgeons with corticosteroids and, in many cases, this relieves the itching, hence the animal rubs less and the inflammation – which is largely self-inflicted – subsides.

Calamine lotion is a useful dressing to apply and may prevent spreading of the condition, especially if used in the early stages.

NETTLERASH – More properly referred to as urticaria, this diseased condition does, in fact, resemble a nettled skin. Elevated plaques of varying size appear on the surface of the body. Sometimes these are all over the horse, at other times they will be confined to localized areas. Itching may or may not be present. Most commonly, the cause is eating something that has not 'agreed' with the animal. There is a local release in the skin of a substance that is chemically akin to the poison in nettles and causes a similar rash. Treatment consists of removing the cause of the trouble by giving a purgative and combating the irritant by administering drugs called antihistamines. As this therapy, although specific, is not without danger, the best first aid is to give a bran mash with about ½ lb. Epsom salts in it.

CRACKED HEELS AND MUD FEVER – These two conditions differ only in the parts of the body that are affected. Mud fever affects the legs and under the belly while cracked heels is a condition of the back of the pasterns. Both are a form of eczema, and both can be very trying to owner and horse and difficult to eradicate.

As the condition is much more prevalent in some parts of the country than others, and as it is most common when the skin has been caked with mud, it is generally regarded as due to some irritant in the soil. White-haired skin is predisposed to cracked heels, and often when a horse has limbs of different colours it is only the white ones that are diseased. It has been suggested that this is because the white legs are washed more often and that the condition arises through imperfect drying, but it seems more likely that white skin offers less resistance to the chapping. Whatever the basic cause, washing and imperfect drying commonly lead to the disease.

Affected parts become sore and covered with a tenacious discharge. In the heels deep painful cracks appear.

Effective prevention is sometimes achieved by coating the heels and under the belly with petroleum jelly or lanoline before taking the horse out.

Treatment is varied and sometimes ineffective. A simple

one for cracked heels is to wash and dry the legs after hunting, using a chamois leather for the drying to avoid friction. Then coat the leg thickly with bran which has been dried and heated in an oven and cover the whole, while the bran is still hot, with a stable bandage. Hot dry boracic lint may be used instead of the bran.

Cod liver oil ointment and lead lotion are other remedies often most effective, as is zinc oxide ointment.

Cracked heels are liable to recur, especially in horses doing fast work, and heels with thickened skin at the back are always suspect.

Horses liable to mud fever or cracked heels should not be washed after hunting unless treated as above. The mud should be allowed to dry on and be removed by brushing the following day.

GALLS AND SADDLE SORES – Galls are wounds of the skin made by friction; saddle sores are galls or are due to pressure causing a part to become bloodless and so much more easily damaged. This type of sore occurs under some part of the saddlery and reveals itself as a raw, open wound often with some swelling around it. Usually it is very painful. Some saddle sores are attributable to the use of plastic foam numnahs, especially home-made ones. These may cause chemical irritation or interfere with the evaporation of sweat.

Treatment comprises removing the cause and often this means that the horse cannot be worked until the sore has healed. In other cases a change of tack, such as substituting a Balding girth for a flat one, may be enough to relieve the pressure and friction, but care must be taken to ensure that this is really the case, as further rubbing quickly causes much harm. Padding may be utilized according to the site: a felt or plastic sponge numnah may be put on and a piece cut away over the sore.

Once the cause has been removed the sore can be helped to heal by the application of sulphonamide powder or acriflavine emulsion.

A horse in 'soft' condition is especially liable to galls and the application of salt solution (a dessertspoonful of salt to a pint of water) will help to harden the skin.

SITFAST – Sitfast is the name given to a condition in which a piece of skin dies while still attached to the animal, or, as the pathologists say, becomes necrotic. Sitfasts are often associated with saddle galls and the usual cause of the skin death is a lack of blood supply caused by unremittent pressure, as from the cantle of a saddle. The dead piece of skin is firmly attached and generally becomes under-run with pus. A painful lesion develops covered with a piece of dark, dry, leathery skin. Rubbing sulphonamide powder or boracic acid under the skin flap will sometimes overcome any infection, but the attached piece of skin usually has to be removed surgically. The cause of the trouble must, of course, also be removed. Opportunities to relieve the horse's back of continual pressure should always be taken during riding by dismounting when at a halt or, at any rate, by the rider altering his position from time to time to relieve the pressure under the cantle of the saddle.

RINGWORM – Textbooks describe ringworm as a fungoid disease characterized by circular patches, devoid of hair in the centre and with broken hairs at the periphery. The skin in the area is scaly and there is usually some irritation. But each of these symptoms is not always present. The bare areas and broken hairs will be there, surely enough, but often the areas are far from circular and itching is not a constant feature. The disease can take an infinite variety of shapes, and when an outbreak occurs in a stable even the most unlikely looking lesions will sometimes reveal the causal fungus when microscopically examined.

The broken hairs are characteristic and, while the disease can only be confirmed by culture or laboratory demonstration of the fungus on or in the hairs, any place with broken hairs is suspect. In some forms of the disease (those most commonly seen) the application of chloroform to the affected areas will cause the hairs to become white and so facilitate diagnosis. Ringworm is spread by infected animals rubbing against one another, or it can be spread indirectly by grooming kit, tack, and infected walls and posts. The incubation period is one to four weeks. The fungus can also affect man, and care should be taken to avoid infection.

The new hair that grows on an infected place is often lighter in colour than before.

Ringworm is troublesome and difficult to eradicate from a stable. An old and satisfactory treatment is the application of tincture of iodine to the affected parts. It is important to prevent the spread of the disease to other horses in the stable, and grooming kit used on an affected animal should not be used on other horses and should be sterilized, preferably by heat. Drugs that are effective against ringworm and can be given in the food are available and work is now proceeding in the hope of perfecting a vaccine against ringworm, which can be very troublesome in large stables, such as racing or army establishments.

LICE – The louse is the commonest skin parasite to appear on horses (which, by the way, do not suffer from fleas). Lice are usually found on animals at grass towards the end of winter, although they may infest at any time both stabled and unstabled horses. The affected animal is itchy, has a dull coat, is usually in poor condition, and has bare areas where it has rubbed away the hair owing to the itch. Sellers of horses sometimes euphemistically describe lousiness as a 'touch of the frost'.

Both biting and sucking lice are found on the horse. They are small grey or black parasites varying in size from little more than a pin head to as big as a match head. A careful search is necessary to find them in some cases, while in others they are so large and numerous that on grey horses they can be seen from a distance of several yards.

Treatment consists of the application of a louse dressing. Gamma benzene hexachloride is particularly good and can be used either as a powder or, better, as a suspension in water which is applied with a brush. Proprietary brands have instructions for application on the packets. As with ringworm, brushings from infected animals should be collected and burned.

Clipping and singeing will destroy the louse eggs (nits) on the hairs.

WARBLES – Although the ox warble fly is not a normal

parasite of horses, equines are not infrequent hosts. The fly has a complicated life history. The adult looks like a hairy bumble bee and lays her eggs on the hairs of the legs of the host in summer. These eggs hatch into tiny maggots which burrow under the skin and creep through the flesh to the wall of the oesophagus (gullet) where they spend the winter. In the spring they migrate to the subcutaneous tissue of the back where they grow into large maggots, 1 in. long and more than $\frac{1}{4}$ in. in diameter. Each maggot makes a small hole in the skin through which it breathes. When the maggot is mature it works its way through the hole and falls to the ground where it turns into a pupa which eventually develops into the adult fly. While under the skin of the back the maggot forms a painful swelling which may interfere with the fitting of the saddle. Often the maggot becomes surrounded with pus. It is important to differentiate the condition from that of an abscess because hot fomentations, which would benefit an abscess, would kill the grub and aggravate the condition. If circumstances permit it is best to wait for the maggot to mature and leave the host naturally. Skilful manipulation will often remove the maggot before its normal time, but if it is ruptured in this process there may be quite a violent local reaction. Differential diagnosis from an abscess is aided by the discovery of the breathing hole on the top of the swelling.

Chapter 7

THE CIRCULATORY SYSTEM

The heart is a muscular pump that circulates blood to all parts of the body. Without adequate circulation no part can function as it should. According to the tissue involved, suppression of circulation will cause ill effects in seconds or hours. The heart of the horse is a massive organ weighing about 9 lb., and is responsible for pumping some six gallons of blood round the body at a rate of about eight gallons a minute. Compare this flow with that of a petrol pump and it will give an indication of what an efficient pump the heart is. The hearts of racehorses, as one would expect, are larger than the average (that of the famous racehorse Eclipse weighed over 14 lb.). Normally the pulse, which can be felt at the angle of the jaw or on the inside of the forearm, is regular and occurs about 40 times a minute – much slower than the human pulse. The pulse is the swelling of the artery that occurs every time the heart contracts and drives another volume of blood through the arteries.

Assessment of the heart condition is a complicated matter and one needing much experience. Abnormalities of the pulse should always be investigated, although in many cases they are not serious. Irregularities in the heart's action are very common, frequently purely functional in character, unassociated with organic change, and do not interfere with the usefulness of the animal. Disease of the heart was formerly considered uncommon, but recent progress in methods of examining the heart, and lawsuits involving horses with heart trouble, have caused modification of this view. Nevertheless, the average owner would do well not to jump too quickly to the conclusion that his horse has a defective heart. A word of warning, however: heart disease may lead to stumbling and the heart should always be carefully examined if a horse is found to stumble for no apparent cause.

ANAEMIA – Anaemia is a condition in which the blood is deficient in either quality or quantity. Deficiency in quality may be due to an insufficiency of haemoglobin or in a diminution of red blood corpuscles. When the anaemia is general, affecting the whole body, the deficiency of quality or quantity is due to imperfect nutrition, wasting, or direct loss of blood. The first symptoms noted by the owner are usually paleness of the mucous membranes and lack of energy.

When nutrition is imperfect the animal will also be thin and the coat is likely to be harsh and dry. Blood-sucking parasites, such as worms and lice, can also cause sufficient loss of blood as to induce anaemia. Hard work when the animal is anaemic is likely to cause damage to the heart and the cause, therefore, should always be sought and appropriate treatment instituted.

AZOTURIA – This condition is one of a number of diseases that used to be included in the term 'Monday morning disease' because it occurs when a horse is worked hard after a rest on full diet. It is, perhaps, more correctly called *myoglobinuria* for reasons that will shortly be made clear.

When the horse has been fully fed and is then worked the circulation in the muscles is incapable of removing the products of metabolism, which then build up in the muscles and cause great pain. One of these products is called myoglobin, and is red in colour. It is eventually excreted by the kidneys into the bladder, and colours the urine dark brown; hence the term 'myoglobinuria'.

An affected animal will appear quite normal and then suddenly stop and seem in great pain. The affected muscles, usually those of the quarters but sometimes other muscles of locomotion, become hard and tense. The horse has a strained, staring expression and, if forced to move, does so stiffly and with great reluctance.

Treatment consists of getting the animal into a loose box with the least possible walking. A horse box should be used to get it to the stable. Once in the stable a bran mash with Epsom salts in it should be given and the horse thereafter kept without exercise on a low diet of hay and bran. Recovery varies with the severity of the attack and may take from a few days to a few months; or the disease may be fatal. Animals which recover from an attack may have depressions in the skin over the sites of the damaged muscles. These indentations may be small, such as might be made by the pressure of a finger, or larger, sometimes even big enough to take one's fist.

LYMPHANGITIS – This is another member of the 'Monday morning disease' complex, and is also called 'weed' or 'big leg'. Throughout the body of the horse, running along by the side of the veins, are similar vessels known as lymph vessels which convey part of the blood back towards the heart. If the circulation through these vessels fails then the affected part becomes swollen and soggy and when pressed with the finger the dent that is made is slow to disappear because the tissues are 'waterlogged'.

When a horse is worked after rest on a full diet the circulation may be inadequate to remove the lymph from the limbs and one or more of them (most commonly one hind limb) becomes swollen and oedematous. The lymph vessels may appear as cords swelling up beneath the skin, and in severe cases fluid will exude through the skin and dry into hard beads or scabs. Infection may be present and the animal is very lame. Sometimes the leg swells up like a bolster and there is a sharply defined line at the top of the affected limb as if a cord has been tied around it.

Treatment consists of putting the animal on a low diet of hay and bran and giving an opening medicine. Certain drugs which are known as 'scheduled drugs' and can only be obtained through a veterinary surgeon are particularly efficacious in dealing with this disease. Light exercise should begin as soon as the horse can bear weight on the limb.

Horses which have had one attack of lymphangitis are liable to a recurrence.

VERMINOUS ANEURISM – This is a grave condition found in some horses which, usually in foalhood, have been infested with round worms. In the course of their life cycle these worms become larvae in the gut of the horse and burrow through the wall of the intestine into the abdominal cavity. They then migrate to various parts of the body before finally returning to the intestines where they grow into adult worms. During the migratory period some of the larvae in the abdominal cavity enter the walls of the blood vessels and, when their numbers are large, do serious damage to the arteries. The most commonly affected blood vessel is the anterior mesenteric artery, which supplies blood to the intestines. The growth in the arterial wall is called an aneurism and may be as large as an orange. The passage of the blood through the aneurism is impeded or stopped and, consequently, the intestine does not receive an adequate blood supply and its normal function is interfered with. This causes such conditions as generally poor condition, anaemia, diarrhoea and colic despite an adequate supply of food Once formed the aneurism persists, even though the horse may be properly dosed for worm infestation. The aneurism may sometimes be felt through the rectum by an operator with a long enough arm and familiarity with the anatomy of the parts concerned. Many cases never recover, and the diagnosis is confirmed at a post mortem. In other cases, however, given time, rest and nourishing food new blood vessels will develop to take the place of the damaged ones and the animals will slowly recover.

Chapter 8

TUMOURS

Horses are liable to develop many kinds of tumours but the three most common types, and those most likely to be seen by the average owner, are *warts*, *melanomata* (black pigmented growths) and *polyps*.

WARTS – Warts are outgrowths of the skin or mucous membrane and resemble the surface from which they arise. They may be mushroom-like with large tops on a narrow stalk or flat growths only slightly elevated above the skin, or they may be anything between these two types. They vary in size from a pin head up to several inches in diameter. They are liable to become infected with bacteria especially when rubbed, as happens when they occur between the legs or in places where they are chafed by the harness. Normally they are painless, but when infected they may become tender and offensive in odour. It is not unusual for them to grow in masses, especially in the ears.

The cause of the growths is not known for certain. Some of them are believed to be due to viruses. An isolated wart in a place where it is unlikely to be rubbed is of little importance, but when warts occur in large numbers, or in places subject to friction, they must be removed.

Warts with stalks ('pedunculated') may be removed by tying a piece of thread (sterilized by boiling) tightly around the stem. This cuts off the blood supply to the growth, which will shrivel up and drop off in the course of days. If the ligature becomes loose as the growth shrinks then a fresh, tight, one should be applied. This treatment is obviously unsuitable for the flat kind of growth.

Often the warts will die if they are coated daily with castor oil or salicylic acid ointment, but this procedure has to be kept up for a week or two. Larger growths must be cut out under suitable conditions with anaesthesia, either local or, in some cases, general. When warts occur in young horses they sometimes disappear spontaneously. In certain cases a vaccine can be prepared from the warts themselves and injected into the horse from whose growths it was prepared ('autogenous' vaccine); in some instances this treatment is unsuccessful but in others it is spectacular in its effects.

A warning should be given against the cruel and heroic treatments which are sometimes advocated. These include the use of violent caustics such as caustic potash, arsenic or red-hot irons. Not only can they cause much pain but they may fail completely and lead to the unfortunate patient becoming very shy, especially if the warts are inside the ears, in which situation treatment even with mild caustics such as silver nitrate may make the animal extremely head-shy.

MELANOMATA – In grey horses, especially when they advance in age, the black pigment (called melanin) tends to collect in tumorous masses in and under the skin, most particularly around the dock. These masses are of a cancerous nature but they tend, especially in the early stages, to fluctuate in size or even disappear for a time. Although these melanomata, as they are called, are most common in older horses (when the grey of the coat is changing to white) the explanation of their occurrence is not simply that the colouring matter is leaving the hairs and collecting in a mass, for the amount of pigment in one tumour is far, far more than would be required for all the hairs of the body.

There is no specific treatment for this condition, although many cases seem to respond to the injection of spleen extract. Owners of horses which develop this condition are advised to seek professional advice early.

POLYPS – These are growths which have stalks attaching them to the surface from which they arise (therefore they include some types of wart). They are most often seen in the nostrils and in the genital passages of mares. They can be removed surgically, often with only local anaesthesia.

RETENTION CYSTS – Although these are not true tumours, mention may be made of them here. The horse's skin contains many sebaceous glands which secrete a greasy substance on to the surface of the skin. Sometimes the ducts from these glands become blocked; the glands continue to secrete sebum, which cannot escape and which therefore makes the glands swell. A common site for this to occur is in the nostril of the horse where a smooth, rounded protuberance appears. It is not painful and feels doughy when pressed. Large ones interfere with breathing and have to be dissected out under anaesthesia.

Chapter 9

EYES

To give the horse a wide field of vision nature has endowed it with prominent eyes, which are consequently exposed to injury. Nevertheless, effective protection has been provided and it is remarkable how seldom the eyes are harmed by severe outside influences. On the other hand, minor injuries from mild causes are common and, if neglected, can have grave consequences.

Injured or diseased eyes are usually extra-sensitive to light and affected animals should therefore be kept in darkened stables.

FOREIGN BODIES – Foreign bodies, such as grass or hay seeds or pieces of chaff or straw, frequently get into horses' eyes, especially if the old-fashioned, high hay racks are used or if the hay nets are tied up too high. Most such foreign bodies are removed by the animal itself by blinking or by the flood of tears that such a stimulus generates. But if the animal fails to shift the offending object then inflammation starts. The eyelids become swollen and tightly closed, tears run from between the eyelids and when the eyelids are parted by the attendant, often with much difficulty, the awn, if such it be, is found to be partly embedded in the front of the eyeball or stuck in place by the inflammatory exudates. An effective way to deal with this condition is to take a tube of eye ointment, remove the cap and squeeze out about a quarter of an inch of ointment. Then take the tube with the pad of ointment protruding and, working slowly so as not to alarm the horse, press it firmly on the seed. The seed will then adhere to the ointment and can be removed from the eye. This technique is more certain than the use of the corner of a handkerchief or similar cloth and much safer than the use of hard instruments. If the foreign body cannot easily be removed in this way it is wise to seek assistance from a veterinary surgeon who will use a local anaesthetic, specially made for use on membranes such as the conjunctiva, before trying to remove the offending object. Do not delay too long, as each day the irritant does more damage and becomes more difficult to remove.

BLOCKED TEAR DUCT – At the inner corner of each eye there are two small openings, one in each lid, upper and lower, which drain away the tears that constantly flood the eye. These openings lead to tubes which run through the skull and emerge in the nostrils. The nostril openings can easily be seen in a quiet horse: they are on the floor of the nasal passage, just where the pigmented and unpigmented parts of the mucous membrane join. Tears have an important protective function, they are of an antiseptic nature and wash away foreign matter from the eyeball which they lubricate. It is fairly common for these tear ducts to become blocked and the tears then run down the face instead of into the nostrils.

On the cheeks the tears may merely make unsightly streaks or they may cause inflammation of the skin. The most common causes of blockage are particles of sand and mucus. Veterinary surgeons check if the ducts are blocked by instilling a dye into the eye. This is diluted with the tears and, if the passages are clear, runs down and stains the inside of the nostrils; when the ducts are blocked no colour appears in the nostrils.

Treatment consists of inserting a catheter into the duct at the nostril end and forcing the obstruction out with a jet of sterile fluid. The operation, though simple, is not one for the layman to attempt.

CONJUNCTIVITIS – The front of the eyeball is covered with a fine membrane which is continuous with that of the inside of the eyelids. This is known as the conjunctiva and although thin and highly sensitive it is remarkably resistant to injury. The eye may be injured by thorns when the horse is jumping a 'bullfinch', by the careless use of the whip, or by the corner of a rug or surcingle being flung on a horse's back. However, when subject to excessive irritation it becomes inflamed and the condition called conjunctivitis develops. The white of the eye becomes reddened through the ingrowth of small blood vessels, there are tears and the eye may be tightly closed.

First aid consists of bathing the eye with a solution of boracic acid in boiled water (1% solution) or with a proprietary eye lotion. The eye lotion should be used in the same strength as the makers advocate for human use. Eye ointments containing yellow oxide of mercury or sulphonamides should then be applied three times a day.

KERATITIS – When the deeper structures of the front of the eye lying under the conjunctiva are inflamed the condition is known as keratitis. Often this develops as a consequence of conjunctivitis. If neglected it can lead to blindness or serious interference with vision as well as causing much pain. First aid is as for conjunctivitis, but skilled assistance should be summoned.

MOON BLINDNESS – No longer a common ailment of the horse in Great Britain, moon blindness is a type of conjunctivitis or keratitis which recurs at intervals of about a month (hence the name) but it is more properly called recurrent ophthalmia. It presents severe and recurring symptoms which apparently clear up and then return in a few weeks. It may attack one or both eyes and often if only one eye has been affected it is the other eye which displays symptoms on the recurrence. After repeated attacks the shape of the eyelid opening is altered to a triangle. The condition is serious and the gravity is obvious at once as the eyelids are tightly closed, a purulent discharge escapes from between them, the orbit is swollen and the horse is obviously ill. First aid is as for conjunctivitis, but again professional aid should be sought.

The cause of moon blindness is uncertain, but both a virus and a lack of Vitamin B have been blamed. The sources of Vitamin B are vegetables, but mere feeding of vitamin-rich food will not cure the condition, though it may well help to prevent it. If Vitamin B has to be administered it must be given in the pure chemical form in massive doses.

Chapter 10

GENERAL DISEASES

ANTHRAX – This is a contagious disease caused by a bacterium which is very resistant to outside influences and hence can contaminate undisinfected soil and buildings for a long time. Whilst it is most commonly seen in Great Britain in cattle and pigs it can also affect horses and man. Symptoms differ with the species. In the horse it is characterized by loss of appetite, high fever, swelling of the head and neck, and death, or by severe fatal colic. Cattle are perhaps most often affected because the most frequent way in which infection is introduced into this country is in cattle food which has become contaminated in the holds of African boats previously conveying infected carcases and hides. Outbreaks of the disease in cattle are frequently traced back to a particular consignment of cattle food shipped here from abroad. The disease is very contagious and the blood from an infected animal especially dangerous. The disease is a notifiable one and if there is any suspicion of its presence the police must be informed; an enquiry will then be made by a veterinary officer of the Ministry of Agriculture, Fisheries and Food.

Cases which are diagnosed early can be treated but it is not, of course, a matter for home doctoring.

TETANUS – This is another disease that affects most animals and man too. It is common in the horse, especially in certain districts. It is caused by a germ which is resistant to adverse conditions and occurs naturally in the intestines of horses and is therefore present in their dung.

The germ is one that grows best in the absence of air, being one of a group of organisms known as anaerobes. It is, therefore, more likely to grow in a wound which closes at the orifice (a punctured wound) than in a large open wound. Punctured wounds are often found in the foot of the horse, the feet are the most likely parts of the anatomy to be contaminated with dung, so tetanus most commonly ensues from punctured wounds of the feet.

The disease has a long incubation period from a few days up to a month or more and so the wound originally infected has often healed long before the symptoms of tetanus are shown. Under suitable conditions the germs grow and produce a poison which acts on the central nervous system.

The disease is also called lockjaw because of the common symptom of the animal being unable to open its mouth. An affected animal cannot eat and becomes sensitive to slight stimuli such as the clapping of hands or the banging of doors. If the patient is flicked under the chin the head may be jerked up and the haw, or third eyelid, shot across the eye. In other cases the horse will stand with the third eyelid constantly showing. As the disease advances the horse becomes stiff in its movements and then stands rigidly with its forelegs advanced and its hind legs pushed out behind. When the horse is made to back the tail will be raised or extended.

Treatment consists of keeping the animal quiet, feeding on soft feed if the animal is capable of prehension and swallowing, plenty of bedding and a darkened stable. Antibiotics and anti-serum together with tranquillizers will probably be used by the attending veterinary surgeon.

An effective vaccination against tetanus is available which lasts for many months before boosting is needed and serum is also given to prevent the onset of the disease when a wound is detected. Horse owners are advised to have their animals protected in this way. (When an insured animal shows signs of this or any other condition which may be fatal the insurers should be informed. Failure to do so may invalidate any claim that may be made later.)

PURPURA HAEMORRHAGICA – This is an alarming condition that may arise spontaneously or, more commonly, follow some disease such as strangles or influenza. The affected animal is obviously ill. It is unwilling to eat or move and its head becomes swollen. The limbs may also be affected and the tongue purple in colour. Purple-coloured spots known as petechiae appear on the surface of the body and are most readily seen inside the lips, nostrils and eyelids. They vary in size from a pin head to more than an inch across. The disease may be confused with an adder bite on the lip which occurs when horses are grazing on snake-infested land. In either case do not delay by trying to make your own diagnosis but call for expert assistance at once.

NAVEL ILL – Also known as joint ill or polyarthritis, this disease is an infection which enters the foal via the navel and symptoms show within the first few weeks of life. The germs are transported round the body in the blood and settle in the joints, causing painful swellings and lameness and general symptoms of illness. Often the infection is severe enough to kill the animal.

Prevention consists of scrupulous cleanliness and attention to the navel at the time of birth. Modern thought is against tying the navel cord, which instead should be allowed to break naturally and not be cut or tied. It may, however, be treated with iodine solution.

Antibiotics, vaccines and serum are used in the prevention and treatment of the disease, which is much more commonly found in foals which have been dropped indoors than in those born in fields.

An infected foal's life is at stake, and professional assistance should be sought at an early stage.

YEW POISONING – The leaves of the yew plant are fatally poisonous to horses, causing death within a few hours of eating. Yews are common ornamental trees in churchyards and formal gardens, often being made into hedges, and horses will readily eat the growing leaves or hedge clippings. Before turning a horse out into a field, make sure there are no yew trees within reach. Snow may weigh down branches to within reach of hungry horses in a snow-covered field.

Chapter 11

WOUNDS

This is one of the most important chapters in this book for the horse owner; wounds are probably the commonest of all ailments and sensible, simple, early treatment can avert much subsequent trouble. However, for sensible treatment to be given it is a great help to have an understanding of how the flesh heals naturally.

The primary symptoms of a wound are gaping, haemorrhage and pain; pain is felt most in the skin, and injured muscles, tendons, and so on are much less painful than injured skin. Pain is more severe when the wound is contaminated and infection has set in.

An uncomplicated wound will heal naturally in one to two weeks, but complications such as infection, foreign matter or movement of the parts may protract the healing period far beyond this.

If the lips of a wound are close together and there is no infection, fluid from the cut edges will bridge the gap and new cells will grow into this and bind the edges together. If the lips are far apart what is known as granulation tissue will grow up from the bottom of the wound and fill the cavity. When the granulation tissue reaches the level of the surrounding skin it stops forming and the skin grows across from the edges. The new cells of skin do not contain hair follicles and a hairless scar will result. An extensive abrasion may heal under a scab when the exudate dries; eventually when the new tissue has grown the scab will fall off.

When a wound is contaminated with bacteria these will grow in the fluid that has been exuded from the damaged cells. Generally the germs cause only local trouble, making the wound painful and interfering with healing; exceptionally they cause generalized illness. When bacteria are present they cause special cells known as phagocytes, which have the property of 'devouring' the bacteria,to come to the part affected. Other special cells are also released into the wound. These phagocytes containing the bacteria and the other cells form what is known as pus. The presence of pus in a wound indicates that bacteria are present they cause special cells known as phagocytes, which have the property of 'devouring' the bacteria, to heal than an uninfected one, but when all the invading bacteria have been destroyed then the wound will heal over.

If a foreign body is present in the wound it may interfere with healing by carrying bacteria on it, or it may interfere mechanically by irritating the cells.

Much movement of the edges of the wound, as when one occurs in the flexure of a joint, will also interfere with healing as the edges of the wound are pulled apart every time they have joined.

Bearing these points in mind a logical procedure for

dealing with wounds can be worked out. When dealing with a recently inflicted wound these simple rules apply:

1. Stop the bleeding. To the uninitiated haemorrhage often seems much more serious than it is; most bleeding will be stopped spontaneously by the animal's in-built mechanism. Tourniquets are dangerous and are very seldom needed. Usually a bandage over cotton wool applied at the end of treatment will be enough to stop blood loss.

2. Remove contaminants such as dirt and grit. Pick out large offending particles and remove the remainder with a gentle stream of water from a hose or by squeezing water from a wad of cotton wool. Normal tap water contains germs and the final wash should be made with a mild antiseptic solution. Avoid rubbing the wound with the cotton wool as this may cause further damage and is likely to rub bacteria deeper into the tissues. Flaps of skin may form pockets in which dirt and the washing fluid are trapped – empty these gently.

3. After decontamination dry the wound by gentle pressure with almost-dry cotton wool.

4. If the wound is such that the lips can be brought together, apply a dressing such as sulphonamide powder, cover with gauze, cotton wool, and bandage, trying to bring the lips of the wound together. If the wound is gaping, an emulsion such as acriflavine emulsion is better than a powder as it will prevent the gauze sticking to the wound. Protect the whole with a stable bandage. Bandages should be changed daily as there is a tendency for wounded tissue to swell and the bandage to become too tight. Do

not change the dressing unless it has become soggy or offensive. After a few days most wounds heal best if left open. It may not be possible to bandage wounds elsewhere than on the limbs and they must be left open. In the summer they may be protected from flies by sticking a gauze covering in place with petroleum jelly. Bandages prevent excess movement, hold dressings in place, protect from further contamination and flies, but are not essential.

5. If there is any bleeding at this stage it can usually be controlled by putting more cotton wool on the wound and adding another bandage.

6. Above all avoid heroic measures. The wound that heals most quickly is the surgical wound – one that, however extensive, has not been bruised or torn and which is not contaminated, and whose edges have been brought into apposition. No treatment other than prevention of movement which might tear the lips apart will hasten healing. Our aim with accidental wounds should be to make them as near to surgical wounds as possible, and after the initial cleansing this entails minimal disturbance. Too frequent changing of dressings and the constant washing away of healing substances produced by the animal will only delay healing and tend to produce 'proud' flesh.

This is not an appeal for neglect of wounds but for more thorough attention in the first instance and then for giving the natural processes the opportunity to work. The fact that nature is the healer and we are but poor assistants should dominate our thoughts and influence all our actions.

7. Steps should be taken to prevent tetanus infection

in all cases where there is a possibility of it, especially when a wound is deep and punctured.

8. Needless to say, if a horse has to be taken out of work because of a wound, it should be put on a low diet of hay, bran mashes and green food – stop oats and cubes.

9. Extensive wounds which need suturing and in which the deeper structures are involved are best dealt with professionally in the first instance. The veterinary surgeon may use antibiotics in his treatment to prevent infection spreading.

If infection is already present when a wound is discovered a variation in treatment is necessary, and all dirt and pus must be removed by washing. A wet dressing of cotton wool soaked in antiseptic or acriflavine emulsion is then applied under cotton wool and a bandage. This is changed twice daily until the wound looks healthy and the gauze covering is inoffensive, when dry dressings may be substituted. Painful infected wounds are treated with hot kaolin or similar poultices which are soothing and 'draw' the wound. These must be changed every twelve hours.

Constant movement, over-enthusiastic cleansing of a healing wound, the liberal application of so-called healing substances, or the prolonged use of wet dressings and poultices may result in the granulations becoming exuberant and protruding above the level of the surrounding skin. Mild cases can be chemically 'burned' back by applying compresses of 5% copper sulphate solution. More severe cases need surgical interference beyond the scope of this book.

Some types of wound need special treatment.

PUNCTURED WOUNDS – These are made by a sharp pointed object which penetrates deeply through a small hole on the surface. This opening soon closes and may be difficult to find, but the penetrating object may have carried germs deep into the underlying tissues. If these germs are of the kind that grow in the absence of oxygen (anaerobes), severe infection may follow. Such wounds are common in horses' feet due to stepping on nails, and are also caused on the breast by pressing on barbed-wire fences. The application of poultices to such wounds is sound preventive medicine. Once again the need for protection against tetanus is stressed.

LACERATED WOUNDS – These occur when the skin and flesh have been torn, as by barbed wire. Usually there is little bleeding as the edges have been torn and the blood vessels seal themselves. Caught early, thoroughly cleansed and dried, these wounds may benefit from having the edges sutured, which will make for quicker healing and less scarring. Barbed wire can sometimes become wrapped around a leg and if the horse panics and kicks terrible wounds can be inflicted. The writer has seen a horse's leg 'sawn off' in this way.

A lacerated wound may be caused by something bigger than a wire barb, such as the bumper of a motor car, and involve the muscles and deeper tissues. Obviously, this is a matter for professional assistance and the best first aid is to get the horse into a loose box, preferably one with adequate artificial light, and stop bleeding by pressure on cotton wool.

In many cases severe, deep and extensive wounds are

best left without sewing up, or sutures may be used in the early stages merely to close gaps in the wound and be taken out long before healing is complete. It is amazing how enormous wounds are capable of healing without loss of function if they are not interfered with too much. Do not be surprised, therefore, if your veterinary surgeon, after examining a large wound, advises no more treatment than rest and allowing it to heal up from the bottom.

OVER-REACHES – These are wounds on the heels of the forelegs caused by the inner edge of the hind shoes. They are apt to occur with tired horses or when an animal gallops from good going into soft ground; the basic cause is inco-ordination. The wound is usually complicated by dirt being forced in, and there is bruising, too. A flap of skin joined to the limb at its base is usually formed. Treatment consists of cleaning thoroughly, applying a dry dressing and bandaging the flap of skin into place. A crepe bandage is useful if the part to be covered is irregular in shape. If the bandage is left off too soon the flap may be torn away again before it has properly healed.

STAKE WOUNDS – These occur in the hunting field and in accidents involving motor vehicles. Their gravity is often difficult to assess and the skin wound may be slight even when serious damage has been done to vital organs. Not infrequently the tip of the stake breaks off in the depth of the wound and while steps should always be taken to see if this is the case, it is often difficult or impossible to ascertain and it may be wiser to wait and see than to risk further damage by probing.

CHEST WOUNDS – These are dangerous because of the risk of penetrating the lungs. Wounds involving the air passages and the lungs and those inside the junctions of the legs and body may become filled with air. This blows up under the skin and distends the animal's body. This air is usually absorbed in a few days, but when the chest is involved it may point to penetration of the lungs.

NOSTRIL AND EYELID TEARS – They are common and are frequently caused by catching on nails, galvanized iron or spring hooks on tie chains. Caught early they can often be sutured and leave little blemish.

KICKS – Kicks frequently produce innocent-looking wounds on the limbs which take a long time to heal as the tissues have been bruised and infected. There is danger too of what are known as 'star' fractures of the under-lying bone. Such fractures are incomplete, but may cause the bone to give way completely when stressed.

INDEX